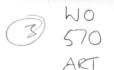
Ultrasound in Anesthetic Practice

Ultrasound in Anesthetic Practice

Edited by

GRAHAM ARTHURS
BARRY NICHOLLS

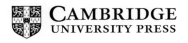

CAMBRIDGE
UNIVERSITY PRESS

CAMBRIDGE UNIVERSITY PRESS
Cambridge, New York, Melbourne, Madrid, Cape Town, Singapore, São Paulo, Delhi

Cambridge University Press
The Edinburgh Building, Cambridge CB2 8RU, UK

Published in the United States of America by Cambridge University Press, New York

www.cambridge.org
Information on this title: www.cambridge.org/9780521716239

First published 2009

Printed in the United Kingdom at the University Press, Cambridge

A catalogue record for this publication is available from the British Library

Library of Congress Cataloguing in Publication data
Ultrasound in anaesthetic practice / edited by Graham Arthurs and Barry Nicholls.
   p.   ;   cm.
Includes bibliographical references and index.
ISBN 978-0-521-71623-9 (pbk)
1. Diagnostic ultrasonic imaging.   2. Anesthesiology.   I. Arthurs, G.   II. Nicholls, Barry.
[DNLM: 1. Ultrasonography.   2. Anesthesia – methods.   3. Anesthesiology.
4. Clinical Medicine – methods. WN 208 U4746 2009]
RC78.7.U4U4465   2009
616.07'543 – dc22   2008037145

ISBN 978-0-521-71623-9 paperback

Contents

Contributors

Vishwanath Acharya MRCP FRCR
Consultant Radiologist
Kettering General Hospital
Kettering
UK

Graham Arthurs OBE MB ChB FRCA FFPMFRA MEd
Consultant Anaesthetist
Maelor Hospital
Wrexham
UK

Owen Arthurs MA MB BChir PhD MRCPCH
SpR Radiology
Cambridge University Hospital NHS Foundation
  Trust
Cambridge
UK

Andy Bodenham FRCA
Consultant Anaesthetist
Leeds General Infirmary
Leeds
UK

Dennis Ll. Cochlin MB BCh FRCR
Consultant Radiologist
University Hospital of Wales
Cardiff
UK

Trevor Frankel BSc AVS
Chief Vascular Scientist
North East Wales NHS Trust
Maelor Hospital
Wrexham
UK

Philip Haslam, MB BS MRCP FRCR
Consultant Interventional Radiologist
Freeman Hospital
Newcastle-Upon-Tyne
UK

Geoff Hide MB BS MRCP FRCR PgDip Clin Ed
Consultant Musculoskeletal Radiologist
Freeman Hospital
Newcastle-Upon-Tyne
UK

Patrick Hill MA CSci MIPEM
Consultant Clinical Scientist
Glan Clwyd Hospital
Rhyl
UK

Tom Ingram MB ChB MRCP
SpR Cardiology
University Hospital of Wales
Cardiff
UK

Stephan Kapral MD
Professor of Anesthesia and Intensive Care
 Medicine
Department of Anaesthesia and Intensive Care
Medical University Vienna
Vienna
Austria

Robert Kong MBBS FRCA
Royal Sussex County Hospital
Brighton
UK

Chandra M. Kumar MBBS DARCS FFARCSI MSc FRCA
Professor of Anaesthesia
The James Cook University Hospital
Middlesborough
UK

Peter Marhofer MD
Professor of Anesthesia and Intensive Care
 Medicine
Medical University Vienna
Vienna
Austria

Barry Nicholls FRCA
Consultant Anaesthetist
Musgrove Park Hospital
Taunton
UK

John Oram FRCA DICM
Consultant Anaesthetist
Leeds General Infirmary
Leeds
UK

David Parker FHFA FRCP FRCR
Consultant Radiologist
Maelor Hospital
Wrexham
UK

Sapna Puppala MRCS FRCSEd, FRCR
Consultant Cardiovascular and Interventional
 Radiologist
Leeds Teaching Hospital NHS Trust
Leeds
UK

Alice Roberts MB BCh BSc
Senior Teaching Fellow
University of Bristol
Bristol
UK

Steve Roberts FRCA
Consultant Anaesthetist
Royal Liverpool Children's Hospital
Liverpool
UK

Henry Skinner FRCA
Consultant Anaesthetist
Nottingham University Hospital NHS Trust
Nottingham
UK

Julian Skoyles FRCA
Consultant Anaesthetist
Nottingham University Hospital NHS Trust
Nottingham
UK

William Taylor M.Obst, FRCOG
Consultant Gynaecologist and Obstetrician
Maelor Hospital
Wrexham
UK

Amy Walker MB, ChB, FRCA
Clinical Research Fellow in Anaesthetics
Birmingham Children's Hospital
Birmingham
UK

Preface

The aim of this book is to provide a practical introduction to medical ultrasound. A few years ago we searched in vain for a book that would give the clinician an introduction to the use of ultrasound in clinical practice. There were many specialist books but no easy to read book that told a trainee or clinician about all the possible uses of ultrasound, what they could learn to do for themselves, and when they should ask others to help. As we explored the subject, we realized that ultrasound is both complicated to understand properly and yet simple to use in practice. In all, we have identified 12 aspects of medical practice in which ultrasound has a part to play. We approached clinicians who are experts in their fields to write a well-illustrated guide to the use of ultrasound.

Clinical ultrasound involves identifying normal and abnormal patterns. We felt that the best way of helping the reader to identify these patterns was to present as many ultrasound scans as possible. This has been made possible by the use of a series of PowerPoint presentations on the accompanying DVD.

The combination of a text book with a DVD combines the best of both educational tools. We hope that the reader will study the text but at the same time view the illustrations on their laptop. In this way the images are reproduced nearer to their original quality. The images will also be larger than possible in any printed text. The video clips show movement, such as the action of the heart, in a way that cannot be achieved in an ordinary text book.

While the first ultrasound was used clinically about 50 years ago, it is the rapid development of micro-computer technology in the past 10 years that has brought ultrasound into everyday clinical practice. It is likely that within the next 10 years, portable ultrasound devices will be carried by all clinicians as they carry a stethoscope or laptop today. We hope that this book will be of help to many students, trainees and practitioners who need to know what this technology can and cannot do. There are also mature clinicians, like ourselves, who have not been brought up with ultrasound, and we hope they will find this a useful way to update their knowledge.

The objective that was set each author was to produce an introduction to their specialist area; to explain what ultrasound can and cannot do; to give practical guidance on how to obtain the best results; to encourage the greater but safer use of ultrasound; and to indicate when to seek further help.

In any multi-authored book, it is inevitable that there will be some overlap between the presentations. These have not been edited out, as each author wrote their chapter as a stand-alone text. Reading more than one explanation of the same subject can also aid understanding.

We are very grateful to all the authors for their efforts, to Tony Bailey and Dr. Alice Roberts for drawing the illustrations, and to the staff at Cambridge University Press for bringing the whole to a successful conclusion.

Graham Arthurs
Barry Nicholls

Chapter 1

Principles of medical ultrasound

GRAHAM ARTHURS, PATRICK HILL
AND TREVOR FRANKEL

Overview

This chapter provides an introduction to the ultrasound process for trainees in anesthesia and other specialties as well as medical students and clinicians not already familiar with this science. It covers the science of what ultrasound is in order to explain what it can do well, where its limitations lie, and how to obtain the best image. It explains the issues which underpin good ultrasound technique, and which inform judgments of what the trainee can achieve and what to do when imaging is challenging and specialist help is required.

Imaging basics

The basic process underlying all types of imaging is simple. It involves mapping out the anatomy or physiology of tissues and organs by seeing how they modify some form of energy provided to them. This can be summarized as three stages of energy transmission, interaction, and reception of the returned energy.

Energy of some form is transmitted into the body. The tissues of the body interact with this energy, and modify it in some way. The modified energy (signal) is then received, and the changes made in the transmitted signal are processed to work out what has happened to the signal on its journey. Finally, these changes are interpreted into clinically useful information about the form and function of the tissues. A clinical image is then made as a map that sets out the information about the physical properties of the tissues. This should bear a clinically useful relationship to either the anatomy or physiology of the tissues in question.

To understand the capabilities and the limitations of an imaging modality, we need to understand the nature of the energy which is being used to interrogate the body, and the nature of its interaction with the different tissues.

Background history: first steps to the piezo-electric effect

Ultrasound is one of the most useful applications of physics to clinical practice. Clinical examination and tools such as the stethoscope only examine the organs through the skin, and require the clinicians to deduce what lies beneath. Ultrasound goes one step further and looks through the skin to measure the size of organs, to detect abnormalities, and, if they move, function and blood flow can be assessed.

Scientific interest in sound started in 1826 when Jean Daniel Colladon first used an underwater bell to determine the speed of sound in water. High-frequency sound, which is not audible to the human ear, was first demonstrated by Lazzaro Spallanzani

Ultrasound in Anesthetic Practice, ed. Graham Arthurs and Barry Nicholls. Published by Cambridge University Press.
© Cambridge University Press 2009.

when he showed that bats navigate by emitting and detecting high-frequency sound.

The ability to generate high-frequency sound waves artificially began in the 1880s with the discovery by the Curie brothers, Pierre and Jacques, that quartz crystals produce an electrical potential when pressure is applied to the crystal. Later work showed that the reverse effect of applying an electric voltage to quartz crystals produced a pressure wave. This was the *piezo-electric effect*, which is the cornerstone of producing ultrasound waves.

Early practical applications of sound: "ultrasound is echoes"

The first SOund Navigation And Ranging device or SONAR (Figure 1.1) emitted a pulse of low-frequency pressure waves under water. This is reflected off the first solid object it meets, such as an iceberg or submarine. This echo is detected, and the time delay between the outgoing pulse and the echo is measured. The distance to the reflector is then easily calculated from the speed of the pressure pulse and the time taken to go out and return.

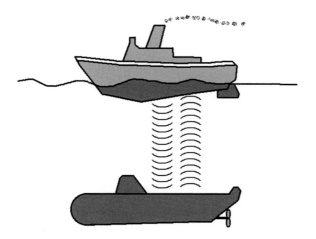

Depth ∝ Time - for signal to return

Figure 1.1 Sonar to determine distance. A single pulse is used.

The same principle of reflection of an energy wave is used in RAdio Detection And Ranging, or RADAR, which uses electromagnetic waves that pass easily through air. Ultrasound waves are pressure waves and so they do not pass well through air, as is seen if ultrasound is applied to the chest to examine the lung, or there is an air gap between an ultrasound transducer and the application site on the body.

An important early scientific application of ultrasound in the 1950s was to detect flaws in the metal plating of battle ships and tanks. The technology that was in use in the shipyards of Glasgow led directly to the first use of clinical ultrasound in obstetrics and gynecology. Ian Donald used this metal flaw detector technology to identify an ovarian cyst and successfully remove it. The fact that it had previously been diagnosed as an inoperable cancer made clinicians take the technology seriously (*Lancet*, 7 June 1958, "Investigation of abdominal masses by pulsed ultrasound"). In the 1960s, Donald turned his attention to measuring the size of the fetal head, and to detecting fetal abnormality, multiple pregnancy and placenta previa.

In the 1950s, in the USA, ultrasound was being used clinically to detect breast pathology.

Intracranial use was attempted but, as we know now, sound waves hardly pass through the bones of the adult cranium. The only present-day use of intracranial ultrasound is in diagnostic neonatology, when the beam can be directed through the open fontanelles.

An early attempted application of high-frequency pressure waves in medical treatment used ultrasound as a form of energy that converts to heat in the body tissues. Many unsubstantiated benefits were claimed for this effect.

Early ultrasound apparatus was large and cumbersome. The patient was surrounded by water in a large tub to enable a good interface between the source of ultrasound and the skin. With the discovery of better piezo-electric materials, starting with lead zirconate–titanate (PZT) in 1954, it became possible to use much smaller transducers, which could be mounted on articulated arms, and applied to the skin. This was much more convenient than the earlier water baths in which patients were immersed. The early transducers operated at the relatively low frequency of 2.5 MHz.

Characteristics of medical ultrasound

By the early 1980s, the ultrasound community agreed to use 1540 m/s as the standard speed for ultrasound in soft tissue in human diagnostic work. The white on black image was adopted as being easier on the eye than black on white.

The development of real-time scanning devices has depended on increasing the rate of the transmissions and reception of the ultrasound waves and reducing the time taken for the interpretation of an ever increasing number of signals. This has been accomplished by increasing the number of transducers that make up the beam.

Faster, high-definition and smaller, portable scanners became possible with the development of the microprocessor chip 4004 in 1971. Its successor, the 8008 chip made by Intel, contains 3300 transistors. The smallest modern ultrasound device has at least 40 Pentium microprocessors making over 20 billion operations every second. Ultrasound devices will become smaller and the images better as the size of the microprocessors reduces, allowing more to be built into a smaller space.

The physics of ultrasound
Sound energy

Sound is energy in the form of a push–pull pressure wave that is propagated in a longitudinal direction. It is a wave in the same way that wind blows over a corn field. The ears of corn move forward and backwards but the roots of the corn do not move forward. Or like a seismic wave passes through the Earth and the Earth stays in the same place. It is a mechanical wave involving physical, oscillating motion, as the medium is temporarily squeezed to high pressure and stretched. The mechanical energy displaces molecules that press against adjacent molecules and so pass the energy on to the adjacent molecules. Each molecule in turn returns to its original position to be compressed by the next wave of increased pressure. The pressure recorded in ultrasound waves can be as high as 10 times atmospheric pressure, but it is a transient change.

The sound wave is characterized by frequency, wavelength and speed. The maximum speed at which the pressure or sound wave passes through a substance depends on the physical properties of the substance. A sound wave cannot travel through a vacuum, where there is no medium or molecules to compress and stretch. The wave motion can be viewed in terms of packets of matter (masses) which must be accelerated, and "springs" which must be compressed and stretched. It follows that the density (mass per volume) and the stiffness of the material are the key physical properties of the medium for ultrasound transmission. The frequency (f) is the number of waves in one second. The wavelength (λ) is the distance between successive high pressures (Figure 1.2).

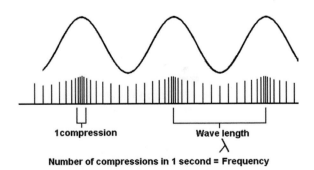

Figure 1.2 Ultrasound wave.

The frequency and speed of sound waves

Frequency is quoted in hertz (Hz). 1 Hz = 1 cycle per second.

The audible frequency range for the human ear is approximately 20 Hz–20 kHz. With age, the sensitivity to higher frequencies in this range is lost. Audible sound waves are transmitted through air at a speed of 330 m/s.

Ultrasound has a frequency above 20 kHz. Frequencies in the range of 1 000 000 Hz (1 MHz) to 20 000 000 Hz (20 MHz) are used for clinical ultrasound.

In this range of frequencies ultrasound is transmitted relatively well through the soft tissues of the body, at a speed of about 1540 m/s, which is the accepted standard for clinical use.

1 Hz = 1 hertz = 1 cycle per second

1 kHz = 1000 hertz = 1000 cycles per second

20 Hz to 20 kHz is called the audible frequency range.

Ultrasound has a frequency above 20 kHz

Clinical ultrasound is in the range of 1–20 MHz.

1 MHz = 1 000 000 hertz = 1 000 000 cycles per second

The time taken from one high-pressure peak to the next high-pressure peak is known as the Period (T). $T = 1/f$.

The speed of the sound wave is determined by the physical properties of the substance or organ it passes through.

The speed $c = \sqrt{(B/\rho)}$

where B is the stiffness (Bulk Modulus) and ρ is the density of the organ.

The typical speed of sound for the different soft tissues of the body is

- Liver   1580 m/s
- Muscle   1575 m/s
- Blood   1570 m/s
- Water   1480 m/s
- Fat   1430 m/s

In order to allow manufacturers to produce medical ultrasound devices that will give comparable images, all devices use a common speed of 1540 m/s, as a working average typical of soft tissue. As we have noted, ultrasound is an echo-ranging technique, and we rely on knowing the speed of the ultrasound to calculate the range correctly. It is important to note that the actual speed of ultrasound varies with tissue type. For example, this means that the thickness of a fat layer will tend to be slightly overestimated, because the actual speed is less than the average speed assumed by the scanner.

In general, ultrasound will be partly reflected at interfaces where there is a change in speed. The bigger the change, the more completely the ultrasound is reflected, and the less is transmitted into the second medium. Thus an interface between air and soft tissue is highly reflective (in either direction), as is an interface between bone and soft tissue.

Speed of sound in other media:

- Air   330 m/s
- Lead   1240 m/s
- Bone   2800 m/s
- Skull bone 4080 m/s
- Aluminum   6400 m/s

Wavelength

The wavelength (λ) is the distance between two high pressures in the sound wave. A simple equation relates speed, wavelength, and frequency.

$C = f\lambda$ (speed = frequency × wavelength)

As we have seen, the speed is a constant for a given medium. This means that the frequency and the wavelength are *inversely* related: i.e. a high frequency produces a small wavelength.

So the wavelength of ultrasound with a frequency of 3 MHz and a speed of 1540 m/s is 1540 m/s divided by 3×10^6 s = 0.0005 m = 0.5 mm

2 MHz ultrasound has a wavelength of 0.7 mm

1 MHz ultrasound has a wavelength of 1.5 mm

The wavelength is important because it is the theoretical limit for *spatial resolution*. In other words, the smallest details that can be interrogated are of the same order of size as the wavelength used. The better the spatial resolution, the better the device is able to distinguish two points that are close together. In soft tissues, wavelengths of less than 1 mm are used, at 2 MHz the wavelength is 0.77 mm. This means that this ultrasound beam might be able to distinguish two points that are 1 mm apart, but will see two points that are only 0.5 mm apart as a single point, not as two points. Shorter wavelengths are related to increasing frequency. Therefore high resolution demands high-frequency ultrasound.

Fundamental properties of medical ultrasound:

- Speed 1540 m/s
- Typical frequency $f = 3$ MHz
- Typical wavelength $\lambda = 0.5$ mm

Generation of the ultrasound wave

The probe that makes contact with the patient contains a large number of individual transducers (Figure 1.3). At least 128 are present in a wide-aperture device, arranged in a line called an *array*. Each transducer has a dual function: it both transmits and receives pulses of ultrasound. It creates and sends out a short burst of perhaps three ultrasound pressure waves and is then silent until it detects those waves returning. This is referred to as pulsed ultrasound. A small group of transducers are activated in turn to emit at the same time followed by another group. In this way, some part of the probe head is always emitting or receiving.

Piezo-electric effect

In order to build up a real-time image, it is necessary to emit and receive many signals in a short period of time. Pierre and Jacques Curie found that a crystal of quartz changes shape when an electric charge or voltage is applied across the crystal. Conversely, when pressure is applied to the crystal, it changes its shape and an electrical charge is created. This two-way process of an electrical charge causing a change in shape that produces a pressure wave, and pressure causing an electrical charge that can be measured, is known as the *piezo-electric effect*. Using this piezo-electric effect, the emitted ultrasound signal is produced by applying an electrical charge to each individual transducer, and the returning pressure wave distorts the transducer to create an electrical charge which can then be processed to create an image.

The sensitivity of the transducer has been increased by replacing early quartz crystals with powdered ceramics such as lead zirconate–titanate, or with plastics such as polyvinylidene difluoride. The sensitivity of each transducer is then increased by polarizing the molecules by heating and then applying a voltage until the mixture cools and solidifies. The poles of the molecules are now lined up to give a maximum change in pressure or current (Figure 1.4, on DVD).

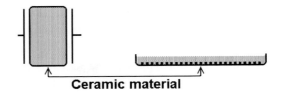

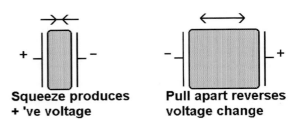

Figure 1.3 Piezo-electric transducer.

Care of the probe

The transducer elements and the probe casing tend to be very brittle and easily damaged if dropped. As we have seen, a typical probe contains many small transducer elements, and each of these must be wired separately. There are many wires leaving the probe, which can be easily damaged by rough use. This happens particularly when scanners are moved between rooms and cables are easily crushed against door frames.

The probe must not be heat-sterilized as this will reduce the polarization and weaken the bonding materials that hold the transducers in place (Figure 1.4a, on DVD).

Refinements in transducer production

Each transducer has a particular frequency at which it will convert electrical energy to sound waves, and vice versa. This is the resonance frequency, which is mainly dependent on the thickness of the transducer element. The thinner the element, the higher the frequency that it can produce.

In practice, the emitted wave is not a single frequency, but a spectrum of frequencies. The number of frequencies is reduced by forming multiple matching layers on the surface of the element. These layers also provide good sound transmission between the transducer and the soft tissues over a range of frequencies.

Modern transducers are constructed of piezoelectric materials that have similar acoustic impedances to that of soft tissue so sound is not lost by reflection at the interface between soft tissue and the transducer.

Real-time scanning

Probe heads with many individual transducers assembled in a line (array) and increased processing speed led to the development of fast B-mode scanners or real-time scanners. The images are updated very quickly to allow the investigation of body movement, such as breathing movements in the fetus.

Weak echoes

A good image requires a good echo. This means that to achieve a good echo, as much of the energy emitted as possible must return to the detector. The image is presented as a gray scale, with strong echoes as white and no echo as black.

Various processes lead to a loss of the energy of the emitted waves and a weaker wave returning to the detector. Collectively, these processes are known as *attenuation*. When the energy wave meets an interface between two tissues, the beam is either reflected, refracted or scattered into many directions. As the ultrasound wave passes through any tissue, *absorption* occurs as sound energy is converted to heat.

The strength and quality of the returning beam is affected by:

- focus and resolution
- acoustic impedance – reflection and refraction
- speckle
- attenuation: scatter and absorption
- artifacts

Focus and resolution

The image of an anatomical feature is built up from a series of points or reflectors which have reflected the beam. In order to get an accurate image of all the points in the tissues from the reflected ultrasound beam, the beam needs to be adjusted to focus at the depth of the points under investigation and have good lateral and axial resolution.

Focus

The ultrasound beam is divided into three zones. (1) The near or Fresnel zone, in which the beam is becoming narrower. (2) The focal zone, in which the beam is narrowest. (3) The far or Fraunhoffer zone, in which the beam widens out. The depth of the tissue under examination should be in the focal zone. In the far zone, resolution is reduced, and it becomes less likely that two points that are close together and at right angles to the beam will be distinguished from each other. Such objects are more likely to appear as a single point.

Lateral resolution is the ability of the beam to distinguish two points that are at right angles (perpendicular) to the beam. If several, close-together points are perpendicular to the beam, then a broad beam will see them as one point. A narrow beam is required for good lateral resolution (Figure 1.5). Lateral resolution is also aided by focusing this narrow beam to the depth of the point which is being examined.

Axial resolution relates to the distance between two points in the path-line of the beam. If two points are close together and in the line of the beam, the scanner needs to be able to separate the distances, which are measured as differences in timing of the echo delay. The ability to separate two points, or axial resolution, depends on the pulse duration (*PD*).

$$PD = N \times T$$

where N = number of cycles in the pulse (often three) and T is duration of each wave or the wave period. The wave period (T) in microseconds (μs) = 1/frequency (f) in MHz

So PD in μs = N/f (MHz)

If the frequency is 3 MHz and the number of cycles in the pulse is 3, the pulse duration is 1 μs. If the fre-

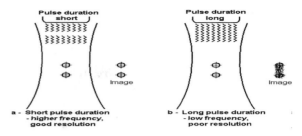

Pulse duration short

Figure 1.6 Axial resolution.

quency is 15 MHz, then the pulse duration is 0.2 μs. It can be seen that, as a rule, the higher frequency (small λ) gives a shorter pulse duration, which leads to better axial resolution. A lower frequency leads to the possibility that two close points in the line of the beam will not be seen as separate points (Figure 1.6, axial resolution).

Contrast

To be distinguishable, two materials should have dissimilar ultrasound characteristics. Contrast resolution can be a problem when two tissues have similar echo intensities. This problem can usually be resolved by adjusting scanner and display monitor settings, and identifying structural patterns in the tissues such as between nerve and muscle (Figure 1.7, on DVD).

Acoustic impedance

When the ultrasound wave meets a change in resistance or impedance at the interface between two different tissues, a part of the wave energy is reflected back to the transducer while part of the wave moves into the next tissue (Figure 1.8, on DVD). This ideal reflection only applies if the beam meets the interface at right angles. The amount of energy reflected at an interface depends on the acoustic impedance of the two tissues. Each tissue has its own acoustic impedance (Z), which is equal to the density (ρ) of the tissue multiplied by the speed of sound (c).

$$Z = \rho c$$

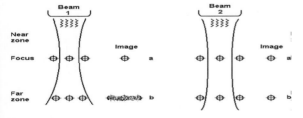

Figure 1.5 Lateral resolution. The clearest image is seen when the beam is narrow and is focused at the depth of the object.

The strength of the signal reflected back when the sound wave moves from one substance to another depends on the change in acoustic impedance. A substance with high acoustic impedance is a good reflector of sound.

Tissue impedances are measured in rayls. 1 rayl = 1 kg/(m² s)

Fat 1.34×10^6 rayl
Water 1.48×10^6 rayl
Liver 1.65×10^6 rayl
Blood 1.65×10^6 rayl
Kidney 1.63×10^6 rayl
Muscle 1.71×10^6 rayl

The difference in impedance is not great between these tissues, and so most of the energy will pass through. However, there is a significant impedance difference between these tissues and Bone 5.6×10^6 rayl and Air 392 kg/(m² s), which means that most of the energy is reflected back at interfaces with bone and air.

A measure of the amount of reflected ultrasound is given by the ratio (R) of the reflected to the incident intensity known as the Intensity Reflection Coefficient (R).

The Intensity Reflection Coefficient $R = (Z_2 - Z_1 / Z_2 + Z_1)^2$ for normal incidence where Z_1 relates to the first tissue and Z_2 to the second tissue.

Consider as an example the interface between fat and kidney.

$$R = (\text{impedance of fat} - \text{impedance of kidney}/$$
$$\text{impedance of fat} + \text{impedance of kidney})^2.$$
$$R = ((1.63 - 1.34) \times 10^6 \text{ rayls}/(1.63 + 1.34)$$
$$\times 10^6 \text{ rayls})^2 = (1.63 - 1.34/1.63 + 1.34)^2$$
$$= (0.29/2.97)^2 = 0.01.$$

This coefficient R is small, meaning that only 1% of the sound energy is reflected back at this interface, and 99% is transmitted. A similar low coefficient can be calculated for all soft tissue interfaces. The interface between soft tissue and air has a high ratio and virtually 100% of the sound wave is reflected at this interface.

Reflection, anisotropy (Figure 1.9) and refraction (Figure 1.10, on DVD)

If the wave hits at any other angle than a right angle, some waves will be reflected at an angle that does not return them to the transducer, and some will be *refracted* as they pass into the next tissue.

The angle of the incident beam is θi, the reflected beam is θr, and the angle of refraction is θt.

The amount of refraction is given by Snell's law.

C_1 is the speed of sound on the incident side and C_2 is the speed of sound on the other side of the interface.

$$\sin \theta t / \sin \theta i = C_2/C_1$$

Reflection and refraction occur as many organs do not have flat, plane surfaces and in particular the reflected echo will be weakest at the edges of round organs such as the kidney.

Anisotropy. A small change in the angle of the transducer in relation to the organ being examined can dramatically reduce the amount of the beam reflected back to the transducer. So when the beam is aimed at the center or flatter surface of the kidney, much of the beam is reflected back at right angles. But when the beam is directed at the periphery of the sphere where the surface is curved, or when the organ is made up of layers but the layers

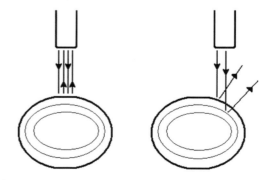

Figure 1.9   Anisotropy.

are not all parallel to the surface, some of the beam is not reflected back to the transducer. This gives a distorted image of the organ with parts appearing whiter or grayer when in reality all the tissue is the same. With smaller structures such as nerves and tendons, the angle at which the probe is held may make the difference between seeing the structure clearly one moment and then it is gone the next moment.

Scatter

When some of the beam hits a small object, the point that makes contact at a right angle is reflected back but most of the wave energy is lost to the surrounding tissues by diffuse reflection in other directions (Figure 1.11). Some of this scattered wave energy can be picked up by other transducer elements, and creates an image of the tissue which does not represent the true structure of the organ. Scatter is a common occurrence and changes the echo-image that comes from within an organ. As a result of scatter, the liver has a homogeneous appearance on a scan, when in reality the organ contains tissues of different detailed structures and echo responses, which are not resolved.

Regions of increased scatter compared to surrounding tissues are hyperechoic and appear whiter. Areas where scatter is low compared to the surrounding tissues are hypoechoic and appear darker. These changes in echogenicity lead to different areas of image brightness that can be used to differentiate between tissues. A hemangioma within the liver is hyperechoic compared to the normal liver, and the fetal lung is hyperechoic compared to the liver.

Rayleigh scatterers, such as red blood cells, are tissues that have a unit diameter that is much smaller than the ultrasound wavelength. A red cell diameter is 8 µm and an ultrasound beam of 5 MHz has a wavelength of 300 µm. This scattering of the sound waves by the red cells causes blood to present an image of a homogeneous tissue. Doppler and color flow studies rely on this homogeneous ultrasound signal scattered by the red blood cells to measure blood flow, even though the individual cells are much too small to be resolved in ultrasound gray-scale imaging.

The amount of Rayleigh scattering increases in proportion to the fourth power of the frequency. However, attenuation also increases with frequency.

Speckle

Speckle is an artifact which gives a grainy appearance to most tissue areas on an ultrasound image. The grain or speckle does not represent a real anatomical feature, but arises due to waves returning from different (unresolved) scatterers adding to or cancelling a signal because of slight differences in echo journey time. Speckle is a form of "visual noise", or "clutter" which generally makes it harder to detect genuine small anatomic features reliably, although it can be used to distinguish homogeneous tissues from fluid-filled spaces (which have no scattering centers). When a lower-frequency (longer wavelength) beam is used, the speckle tends to be more pronounced, and whiter spots appear larger with less black between. The appearance of the speckles depends on the type of tissue, the depth and the transducer characteristics.

Attenuation

As the signal travels deeper into the tissue energy is being lost, because of absorption and scatter (Figure 1.12). So the energy of the echo reflected from deeper tissues will be weaker than the energy

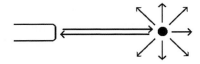

Figure 1.11 Scatter.

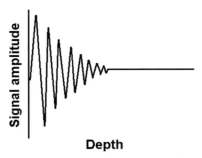

Figure 1.12 Attenuation of signal with depth.

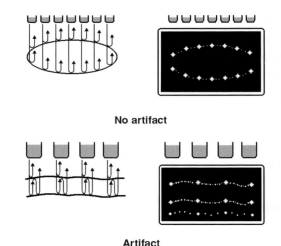

Figure 1.13 Creation of an artifact.

of waves reflected from the superficial tissues nearer to the transducer. This would mean that the deeper picture will be of a different gray image quality when the tissue is actually the same. *Time gain compensation* is used to amplify the signal from deeper tissues to make the image look the same on a gray scale as the signal from superficial tissue.

Artifact

An artifact is an image feature that does not represent a tissue structure (Figure 1.13). One example is a reverberation artifact. This occurs when a returning echo is reflected back into the tissue and then reflected for a second time before returning to the transducer. The returning second signal is counted in time and converted to another depth. So an image is built up of a double (or multiple) structure at greater depth, which is artifact. An example of this is seeing lines in the lumen of the trachea, which represent multiple images of the trachea–air interface.

Which probe?

As we have seen, good resolution generally requires high-frequency ultrasound probes. Unfortunately, high frequencies are more strongly attenuated than low frequencies. Good penetration (maximum working depth) requires a low frequency. This means that there is a compromise to be struck between "depth" and "detail". So the highest

frequency for the depth of the target in the tissue is chosen, e.g. abdomen 3.5 MHz or neck 7 MHz.

A linear array emits linear wavefronts and a rectangular image is created. This probe might be used to visualize the veins in the neck.

A curved array emits signals in a radiating arc. This is useful when the window through which a beam can be sent is small, such as the space between two ribs to examine the heart.

An annular array emits signals all round the circle. This is used in the vagina or rectum.

Terminology of modes

The A-mode (amplitude mode) displays the single echo signal as in SONAR against time. The time for the echo to return is a measure of the depth. This is still used to determine the exact dimensions of the eye, but it is limited by only giving results from single impulses along a single beam.

B-mode (brightness mode) has developed from A-mode. The B-mode image is a two-dimensional (2D) image built up using multiple beam positions and a series of reflected echoes. The image is made up of a number of dots; each dot has an intensity related to the amount of energy being reflected. The B-scan is improved by time gain compensation.

M-mode (motion mode or time-motion mode, T-M) uses a small stationary B-mode beam to examine a moving structure, plotting out how the structure moves with time. An example of this use is to show the movement of the heart wall and valves. The B-mode trace moves across the screen. The display shows reflected depth on the y axis and time on the x axis. The limitation of the M-mode view is that it is along a single axis.

Doppler shift

In 1842, Christian Andreas Doppler described the phenomenon illustrated by listening to a passing train. When the origin of a sound wave is approaching the hearer, the wavelength shortens and the pitch rises. As the origin of the sound goes away from the hearer the sound wave lengthens and the pitch falls. In terms of physics, the approaching waves are compressed and of shorter wavelength, while the receding waves have a longer wavelength. This change in frequency is called Doppler shift (Figure 1.14).

In the case of ultrasound waves, which are being emitted and detected by the same transducer:

- If the object is moving towards the source of the ultrasound then the frequency that was transmitted increases on the return.
- If the object is moving away from the ultrasound source the transmitted frequency decreases on the return.

The Doppler shift frequency is the difference between the frequency of the emitted ultrasound and that of the received echo. By measuring the change in frequency, the direction and speed of movement can be calculated.

In order to assess flow by Doppler shift, the beam should not be at right angles to the flow. This can be proven by considering the equation for the change of frequency given by:

$$f_D = 2 f_0 v \cos \theta / c$$

where

f_D = the Doppler frequency;
f_0 = the transmitted ultrasound frequency;
v = the reflector velocity; and
c = the speed of sound.
Cos θ = the cosine of the angle between the transmitter beam and the reflector pathway. Cosine of $90°$ = 0, so if the beam is at right angles to the flow no Doppler shift will occur. In practice, the perpendicular beam that produces the best B-mode images produces no signal for flow and makes it impossible to measure the velocity of a moving object. An incident angle of between $30°$ and $60°$ with the vessel lumen gives the best angle to estimate the velocity.

The assessment of blood flow is complicated by the fact that blood flow in an artery is not a simple uniform profile. The velocity profile may be parabolic (as in laminar flow), with the maximum flow along the central axis and zero flow at the vessel wall, or almost rectangular as in large vessels such as the aorta, or asymmetrical in a variety of ways.

Doppler devices have developed from simple flow visualization to the assessment of velocity and waveforms and now to color flow mapping, power Doppler and Doppler tissue imaging.

Safety of ultrasound

Ultrasound has been used on vast numbers of patients around the world over four decades, with an excellent safety record, even in sensitive applications such as obstetrics. Very useful summaries of ultrasound safety issues can be found

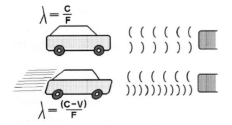

Figure 1.14 Doppler effect.

on the British Medical Ultrasound Society web-site (www.bmus.org). However, it must also be noted that the output power of ultrasound has been increasing in recent years, and it is also possible that there are subtle or transient effects which are not yet fully characterized. Hence a precautionary approach is advised, so that diagnostic ultrasound is only considered safe when used prudently.

There are several mechanisms to be considered by which ultrasound might cause harmful effects: direct mechanical, thermal, and cavitation.

Power values vary widely, but typical values are M-mode 4 mW, B-scan 18 mW, Pulsed Doppler 30 mW and Color Doppler 80 mW. Tests have shown no adverse effects in human tissue exposed to less than $100 \, \text{m W/cm}^2$.

Heat is produced when the ultrasound is atten-uated in the tissue by absorption. Ultrasound pro-duces a measurable rise in temperature in tissue when the beam is of high intensity and used for a long exposure. Any heat produced will normally be lost by spread to other tissues. The key fac-tors are the ultrasound power output, focusing, and time. The worst combination might be for the operator to keep the scan-head stationary, using a non-scanning mode (such as M-mode or spec-tral Doppler, which have a single line-of-sight), and a high-power output setting. Modern ultra-sound scanners are required to display a *thermal index* value, that gives an indication of the tem-perature rise which is likely to be produced by the choice of settings. Some tissues absorb ultrasound more strongly than others, so tissue-specific ther-mal indices are used: TI-b (bone), TI-s (soft tissue), and TI-c (cranium). The usual guidance is to assume that the actual temperature rise could be as much as twice the TI value estimate.

Ultrasound therapy devices have spatial average-time or average intensities of $1000 \, \text{mW/cm}^2$ to pro-duce deep heat.

Intense ultrasound can produce very small gas bubbles, called cavitation, from the gas normally dissolved in solution in the tissues. The bubbles will either oscillate, known as stable oscillation, or grow in size and collapse abruptly producing local micro-explosive effects called transient cavitation. This latter effect is well known in vitro, and provides the scouring effect of dental descalers and labora-tory ultrasound cleaning baths. Modern ultrasound scanners display a mechanical index (MI) value, which gives an indication of the chance of cavitation effects, given the ultrasound parameters selected. In general, the risk is increased by (a) the presence of seeding bubbles (such as gas-filled ultrasound contrast media), (b) increasing power, (c) increas-ing exposure time (particularly with non-scanning ultrasound modes), and (d) lower ultrasound frequencies.

For safe use, clinicians should be familiar with the hazard factors, and how they relate to the scanner settings, and should be careful to limit scans to the minimum time required to gain the desired clinical result.

High acoustic intensities should only be used when the clinical conditions warrant their use.

Where present, the receiver gain control should be set at high and the (ultrasound) power set-ting control should be set at low, and not the reverse. The examination should start with a low-power output and this should only be increased if the maximum received gain does not give a good result or when there is noise and not sufficient penetration.

The operator should avoid holding the scanner in one position on the patient when it is not being used.

Applying the physical principles to the ultrasound controls
The ultrasound controls

In order to create the best possible ultrasound image and minimize the factors listed above that affect the quality of an ultrasound image, ultrasound devices are fitted with several adjustable controls. Most modern ultrasound machines also have *preset* controls for different types of examination. It is important to select the most appropriate preset before commencing an ultrasound examination. The presets are useful for achieving a good general setup for each examination type. In order to obtain optimum image quality, however, it is important to understand how to alter the settings on the machine.

An explanation of the most commonly used controls is given below. This list is not exhaustive and more complex ultrasound machines will have many settings that are not mentioned here. It would be best to refer to the manufacturer's guidelines for more information about these additional controls.

2D B-scan controls

Gain provides overall amplification of all the received echoes. This affects the brightness of the image. Generally the gain is increased for looking at deep structures and decreased for looking at superficial structures (Figure 1.15, on DVD).

Time Gain Compensation (TGC). Weaker signals are received from structures that lie deep and stronger signals are received from structures that are superficial (due to attenuation). The TGC is used to amplify signals from different depths, so that equal amplitudes may be displayed from all depths. It increases amplification with increasing depth. Some machines have several sliding controls to adjust this setting for different depths. Other machines simply have two rotating knobs, which can control the "near" gain and the "far" gain (Figure 1.16, on DVD).

Focus adjusts the imaging depth

Focus adjusts the depth at which the ultrasound beam is focused. Focusing adjusts the ultrasound beam to be at its narrowest at the selected depth. This improves the lateral resolution of the image. The focus depth should normally be set at the level of the tissue to be examined. Some

ultrasound machines have the option of selecting multiple focal zones. Other ultrasound machines do not have the option of selecting focus depth at all. These latter machines usually focus to the center of the image, and thus the region of interest should be positioned in the center of the screen. Use pressure on the probe or the depth control to assist with focusing.

Optimize. This control is used to alter the frequency of a broadband ultrasound probe. This is often set up for superficial, general or deep work. When "superficial" or "resolution" is selected, a higher frequency will be transmitted which will provide better axial resolution. When "deep" or "penetration" is selected, a lower frequency is used which will provide better penetration but lower axial resolution. More complex machines allow greater flexibility in selecting the frequency transmitted by the probe.

Tissue harmonic imaging (THI). This function filters out the low-frequency fundamental components of the ultrasound echoes and uses the second harmonic components to form B-mode images. This helps to reduce reverberation artifact, thus improving image quality (Figure 1.17, on DVD).

Dynamic range. This control alters the range of signal value that a system processes from a scanhead without distortion. A low dynamic range gives a highly contrasted image, which is often better for seeing the wall of a vessel. A high dynamic range gives a lower contrast image, which is often better for detecting changes in soft tissue (Figure 1.18, on DVD).

Dual image splits the ultrasound display in two. This allows a frozen image to be retained on the screen, whilst a real-time image is viewed alongside.

Pulsed Doppler controls. Pulsed Doppler mode gives a trace with velocity (or frequency) shown on the y axis and time on the x axis. Flow towards the transducer is usually represented as a positive velocity value and flow away from the transducer as a negative velocity value.

Gain adjusts the amplification of the Doppler signal. This should be adjusted so that background noise on the Doppler trace is minimal (Figures 1.19a and 1.19b, on DVD).

Scale/pulse repetition frequency (PRF). Increase this frequency when sampling high velocities to avoid aliasing. Reduce it when sampling low velocities to avoid missing very low velocity components (Figure 1.20, on DVD).

Baseline. This control adjusts the level of the "baseline" between positive and negative velocity traces. The baseline can be raised to demonstrate more negative velocity values or lowered to demonstrate more positive velocity values (Figure 1.21a and Figure 1.21b, both on DVD).

Invert. This control switches the displayed direction of flow. For example, a positive direction of flow displayed above the baseline can be inverted so that it is displayed below the baseline (Figure 1.22a and Figure 1.22b, both on DVD).

Doppler beam steering. The angle of the Doppler beam may be steered to assist in achieving the best Doppler shift signal. The best Doppler shift signal is achieved when the flow is interrogated at 60° or less (Figure 1.23, on DVD).

Angle correction adjusts the angle of the Doppler cursor line. The machine uses this angle to calculate the velocity of blood flow. It is therefore important to angle the cursor parallel to the wall of the blood vessel (or the presumed direction of flow) to achieve an accurate calculation of flow velocity (Figure 1.24, on DVD).

Gate size also known as sample volume/sample width. This is the volume in which velocities are sampled. The gate size is usually kept small, to allow for discrete sampling of the velocity profile. It may be useful to temporarily increase the gate size when it is difficult to detect flow (low flow, or excessive vessel movement) or when measuring volume flows (Figure 1.23, on DVD).

Sweep speed adjusts the speed at which the Doppler trace sweeps across the screen. A slow sweep speed will allow more cardiac cycles to be displayed on the screen at any one time. A fast sweep speed will display fewer cardiac cycles on the screen.

Color Doppler

The color Doppler mode brings up a box on the screen. Any changes in frequency detected within the area denoted by this box will be assigned a color (usually red or blue). In practice, this means that blood flow will be demonstrated within this box and shown in either red or blue (depending on the direction of flow). A color wheel or bar on the screen will show which color has been assigned to positive and negative flow directions (Figure 1.25, on DVD).

Gain adjusts the amplification of the Doppler signal from the area shown within the color box. If this is set too high, color "bleeding" will be seen across the vessel walls into the surrounding tissues. If this is set too low, incomplete color filling of the vessel may be seen (Figure 1.26, on DVD).

Scale. Increase this when sampling high velocities to avoid aliasing. Reduce it when sampling low velocities to avoid missing very low velocity components (Figure 1.27, on DVD).

Invert switches the displayed colors for direction of flow. For example, a positive direction of flow displayed in red can be inverted so that it is displayed in blue.

Angle color box. The best Doppler shift signals are achieved when the vessel is at 60° or less in relation to the color box. If the vessel is perpendicular to the color box, poor color filling may result (Figure 1.28, on DVD).

Size of color box. The width of the color box will affect the frame rate. A wide color box will result in lower frame rates.

Power Doppler. Power Doppler maps the density of all moving blood cells regardless of speed or direction. This can be useful in low flow situations (Figure 1.29, on DVD).

FURTHER READING

Cole SEA. *Vascular Laboratory Practice Part 1*. York, IPEM, 2002.

Kremkau FW. *Doppler Ultrasound: Principles and Instruments*. Philadelphia, Saunders 1995.

Zagzebski JA. *Essentials of Ultrasound Physics*. Philadelphia, Mosby, 2006.

Sonosite MicroMaxx User Guide (www.sonosite.com).

Operation Manual for Diagnostic Ultrasound System Application. Toshiba (www.toshiba-medical.co.uk/ultrasound).

www.ob-ultrasound.net/history1.html
www.nelh.nhs.uk/screening/fasp/history.html
forums.obgyn.net/ultrasound
www.aium.org/aboutAIUM
British Medical Ultrasound Society (BMUS) website (www.bmus.org).

ACKNOWLEDGMENT

The authors are grateful to Tony Bailey for the line illustrations.

Chapter 2

Ultrasound to aid vascular access

PHILIP HASLAM

Introduction and controversy.

(1) Internal jugular vein anatomy and the land-mark technique.
(2) Femoral vein anatomy.
(3) The NICE guidelines.
(4) The equipment.
(5) Safe ultrasound internal jugular venous access.
(6) Where ultrasound can be particularly helpful.
(7) When you should call for help.
(8) Conclusion.

Introduction

Central venous lines are inserted for a variety of reasons including total parenteral nutrition (TPN), cytotoxic drug administration, dialysis and fluid administration. It is estimated that approximately 200 000 central venous access procedures are performed annually in the UK [1]. The traditional technique for line insertion is by using anatomical landmarks. The technique is simple, but complications can occur in up to 10%. These complications can be serious and include arterial puncture, pneumothorax, nerve injury and misplacement of the line [2, 3].

Examples of complications

The placement of a large dual lumen dialysis line into the left common carotid artery (Figure 2.1).

This was removed in theater uneventfully and hemostasis achieved with compression.

The unfortunate result of an accidental carotid puncture during attempted jugular line placement (Figure 2.2). The arterial puncture dislodged a plaque/thrombus which caused the large right cerebral infarction. The patient subsequently died.

A large right-sided pneumothorax following right subclavian line insertion (Figure 2.3).

The National Institute for Clinical Excellence (NICE) issued guidelines in 2002 on using ultrasound for central venous access [4]. These guidelines provoked considerable debate, mainly amongst anesthetists.

The vast majority of anesthetists are extremely skilled in central venous access, performing hundreds of such procedures every year. Some have been offended by the guidelines and have taken the approach that the landmark technique is good enough. They argue that the use of ultrasound may lead to loss of skill in the landmark technique, which is the very technique that may be needed in an emergency situation. NICE states that the operator should maintain skills in both techniques.

The various Internet discussion forums have made interesting reading over the last few years. Here are a few examples ranging from the skeptical to the enthusiastic.

Ultrasound in Anesthetic Practice, ed. Graham Arthurs and Barry Nicholls. Published by Cambridge University Press.
© Cambridge University Press 2009.

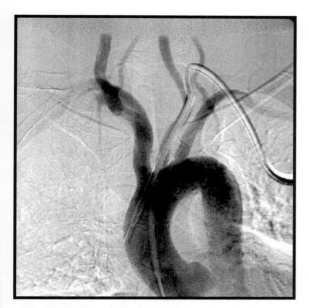

Figure 2.1 A large dual lumen dialysis line placed into the left common carotid artery.

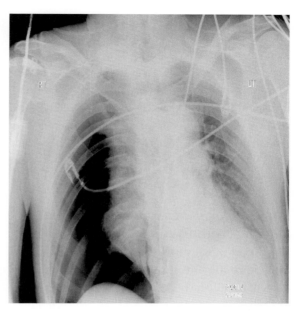

Figure 2.3 Pneumothorax after a right subclavian line insertion.

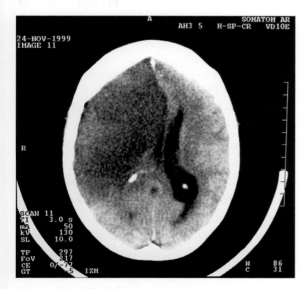

Figure 2.2 Arterial puncture of the carotid artery leading to dislodgement of a plaque causing a right cerebral infarction.

"Not necessary unless problems predicted. Useful skill to have, like everything.

Leave to individual preference as a learning curve occurs with all equipment and we'll create another rod for our own back when unnecessary precautions become expected."

"Used one in anger last night in collapsed major haemorrhage 'obs' patient. Very experienced SpR had already failed and hit the carotid. Landmarks hazy, have to say it worked a treat! Will still teach landmark technique, but not so sceptical of U/S machines."

"I am a fan. Have used them for routine and difficult ones. Made difficult one like taking candy from a baby. For straightforward ones, useful to scan a neck when teaching. Also came across a virgin neck with no RIJ vein and one where patient was so dry that the vein collapsed completely on inspiration... in consecutive cases. If we have the means to 'see in the dark,' I think it is foolish not to BE ABLE to use it. It is after all a procedure that carries risk in terms of morbidity and mortality. It's not to replace existing techniques, but compliment current methods."

The discussions seem to have swayed more towards the latter style of comment, with people now realizing precisely how ultrasound can be of real use in central venous cannulation.

I learned to perform central venous access without ultrasound whilst working as an RMO and SHO in renal medicine in the early 1990s. It was then unheard of to use ultrasound outside of the radiology department. I thought I knew the relevant anatomy and had been taught where to puncture the subclavian vein and jugular vein (both high and low approaches). Nevertheless, I remember numerous occasions when I and more senior colleagues were unsuccessful in puncturing the vein. Since then, as an interventional radiologist I have placed hundreds of venous lines in various different locations and now appreciate the reasons we failed on some occasions. The commonest and probably easiest location for line insertion is the internal jugular vein. I will therefore devote most of the discussion to this vein.

Internal jugular vein anatomy and the landmark technique

This is traditionally performed with the head turned away from the side of puncture. The internal jugular vein usually traverses from posterior to the common carotid artery, to lateral, to anterior as it travels inferiorly in the neck. It is most superficial in the upper part of the neck (Figures 2.4 and 2.5, both on DVD).

High internal jugular vein punctures are performed by palpating the carotid artery and puncturing just lateral to it. The low approach punctures between the two heads of sternocleidomastoid just above the clavicle. The high approach is more risky for inadvertent carotid puncture, whereas the low approach has a higher risk of pneumothorax.

The traditional landmark technique is described as follows in anesthetic teaching (http://www.frca.co.uk).

Use an aseptic technique. The operator should be gowned and wear sterile gloves. The site should be cleaned and draped.

(1) Inject local anesthetic into the center of the triangle formed by the two heads of the sternocleidomastoid muscle and the clavicle.

(2) Introduce a needle whilst aspirating with a 10 ml syringe. Palpate the carotid artery ensuring that the needle passes lateral to it. Direct the needle caudally, parallel to the sagittal plane, at a 30° posterior angle with the frontal plane, aiming towards the ipsilateral nipple.

(3) Once blood is aspirated, cannulate the vein using the Seldinger technique.

(4) The catheter tip should lie in the superior vena cava above the pericardial reflection. Perform check chest X-ray to confirm position and exclude a pneumothorax.

There are several reasons for failure of this method even in experienced hands.

(1) The internal jugular vein may be absent or hypoplastic.

(2) The vein may be stenosed or thrombosed. This is not uncommon in patients who have had previous multiple access procedures, particularly dialysis lines.

(3) The vein may be positioned posterior to the carotid artery.

(4) The vein is compressed and completely collapsed by the finger palpating the carotid artery.

(5) The vein may be compressed by hematoma from previous needle passes.

(6) The vein is collapsed in a hypotensive patient.

FEMORAL VEIN ANATOMY

The femoral vein lies immediately medial to the common femoral artery at the inguinal ligament. It then rapidly comes to lie posterior to the artery within 4 cm of the ligament. This is contrary to traditional anatomical teaching, which suggests that this altered relationship occurs much more distally in the thigh (Figure 2.6, on DVD).

This rapid alteration in the "normal" relationship can lead to failure of cannulation if the access is attempted too distal to the inguinal ligament. The landmarks for the ligament (anterior superior iliac spine to the pubic tubercle) are not easy to find in obese patients and could be missed in an emergency situation.

Another cause of failed femoral vein cannulation with the landmark technique is compression of the vein by the fingers palpating the femoral artery.

THE NICE GUIDELINES

The National Institute for Clinical Excellence issued guidance on the use of ultrasound locating devices for placing central venous catheters in the technology appraisal Number 49 [4]. The authors made the following recommendations.

(1.1) 2D imaging ultrasound guidance is recommended as the preferred method for insertion of central venous catheters (CVC) into the internal jugular vein in adults and children in the elective situation.

(1.2) The use of 2D imaging ultrasound guidance should be considered in most clinical circumstances where CVC insertion is necessary either electively or in an emergency situation.

(1.3) It is recommended that all those involved in placing central venous catheters using 2D imaging ultrasound guidance should undertake appropriate training to achieve competence.

(1.4) Audio-guided Doppler ultrasound guidance is not recommended for CVC insertion.

Other comments include:

"the landmark method would remain important in some circumstances, such as emergency situations. Consequently, the Committee thought it is important that operators maintain their ability to use the landmark method and the method continues to be taught alongside the 2D-ultrasound-guided technique."

There is a patient information leaflet on the NICE guidance which states the following. "If you or someone you care for is going to have a clinical procedure which might involve inserting a central venous catheter (for example, major surgery), you should discuss this guidance with your doctor or nurse."

THE EVIDENCE

These guidelines are based on an analysis of 20 randomized controlled trials, 13 were of real-time 2D ultrasound versus the landmark technique, with the remainder studying Doppler versus landmark technique. Outcome measures included failure rates for first and subsequent attempts, complication rates, number of needle passes and time to successful insertion. The results were pooled for meta-analysis where appropriate.

The analysis found an 86% reduction in failed catheter placements ($p = 0.00001$), 41% reduction in failure on first attempt ($p = 0.009$) and a 57% reduction in the risk of catheter placement complications ($p = 0.02$). Line insertion was on average 69 s faster with real-time 2D ultrasound ($p < 0.00001$).

The evidence is less clear-cut for the subclavian route, with one trial favoring the ultrasound method (55% failure with landmark vs. 8% with ultrasound). However, the operators were relatively inexperienced with both methods. It is likely that these figures would be different in more experienced hands [5].

Ultrasound is also of benefit in femoral vein catheterization. A study by Hilty et al. [6] found a 71% reduction in the risk of failed catheter placement with, on average, 2.7 fewer attempts.

The landmark technique relies on the presence of a patient vein in the expected position. If this is not the case then cannulation is less likely to be successful.

A case series [7] looked at this and also the results of other studies, finding that ultrasound diagnosed between 9% and 20% of patients as having either thrombosed veins or aberrant jugular anatomy.

EQUIPMENT

The rapid pace in the development of microelectronics has seen progressive miniaturization and reduction in cost of ultrasound machines. Most can be bought for between £10 000 and £20 000. Some have the capability of the larger machines found within the radiology department only a few years ago.

A basic machine is all that is required for guiding venous access. Color and pulsed Doppler are not strictly necessary, but color can sometimes be useful to help identify areas of acute (isoechoic) thrombus.

The following list gives some of the desirable or essential features.

(1) Portable, battery-/mains-operated.
(2) Possibility to be stand-mounted.
(3) Robust.
(4) Display easily viewed under ambient lighting conditions.
(5) Linear array probe 5–10 MHz
(6) Low cost.

Sonosite manufacture a range of equipment suitable for portable use ranging from the iLook, Sonosite180plus to the Titan. I have personally used all of this equipment and find the iLook ideal for access work. Some departments will find the larger machines such as the Titan more useful, being capable of a wider range of scanning applications.

(1) The iLook is smaller than the 180 with a shorter battery life (Figure 2.7, on DVD). It is ideal for venous access work, but not well-suited to more demanding tasks.
(2) The Sonosite 180 is fitted with a curvilinear probe (Figure 2.8, on DVD). This probe could be used for venous access, but a linear probe is better. On the contrary, a high-frequency linear probe would be next to useless for abdominal scanning.
(3) The Titan can be removed from its stand. It is a more sophisticated machine and can be used for other types of scanning (Figure 2.9, on DVD).

SAFE ULTRASOUND-GUIDED INTERNAL JUGULAR VENOUS ACCESS

Although the discussion refers to the internal jugular vein, the technique can be adapted for any vein. I would suggest reading through the following method with reference to the picture slides, then watch the video (Figure 2.12, on DVD), jugular vein cannulation.

The initial ultrasound puncture can be made using the standard 19 g needle that is packaged with most access sets. The author uses a Cook micropuncture kit (Figure 2.10, on DVD) for small vessels and patients with difficult access. The advantage is that the initial puncture is made with a 21 g needle which is less likely to cause trauma if misplaced. Figures 2.11 and 2.13 through to Figure 2.18 illustrate the use of the kit (on DVD).

A sterile plastic probe cover should be used with a single use sachet of ultrasound gel to maintain sterility.

(1) The probe can be placed either transversely across the jugular vein or longitudinally. I tend to use the transverse method, as the probe then takes up less room. This is important to obtain a low jugular puncture for tunnelled line insertion just above the clavicle. *It is important to remember that the needle can easily be advanced obliquely through your transverse field of vision and beyond.* This is a common cause of inadvertent carotid/subclavian artery puncture by the inexperienced operator. The needle tip should be kept in direct vision by altering the angle of the probe as the needle is advanced. Scanning longitudinally avoids this problem, but could lead to a higher puncture unless you scan from the side. The needle may sometimes not be seen, but its position can be deduced by the indentation it makes in the soft tissue and on the wall of the vein. It is important to be especially vigilant if the needle is not seen clearly.
(2) Some operators scan the patient before puncture to locate the vein and check its patency. They mark the vein's position, then puncture without ultrasound. This is a perfectly adequate technique in experienced hands, but not strictly within the NICE guidelines.

(3) The needle should be advanced under ultra-sound guidance into the vein and blood aspi-rated with a small syringe. You will see from the video that the vein is easily compressed by the needle, especially if the venous pressure is low. A Trendelenburg position is often helpful to fill and distend the vein. Once the vein is entered, the needle should be flattened so that it is more parallel to the neck. This will make wire advancement easier.

(4) An 0.018 inch wire is advanced through the micropuncture needle into the vein. If there is resistance then the needle tip may need redi-recting, and it may help to scan the wire as you try to advance it.

(5) The 5F sheath and its central stiffener are then advanced over the 0.018 wire.

(6) The stiffener and wire are removed. This leaves the outer 5F sheath in place to insert a 0.035 inch standard wire.

(7) The 0.035 inch wire is inserted. The sheath is removed and the dilators and line can be inserted as normal.

(8) The patient should have a post-procedure chest X-ray to confirm the catheter tip position and to exclude a pneumothorax or a hemothorax. A pneumothorax may appear immediately, but it can be delayed for several hours, so a chest X-ray taken within 30 min can lead to a false sense of security. This is not necessary if the proce-dure was done with additional X-ray screening.

Potential problems with jugular access

(1) The wire will not advance.
  (a) This is often due to the tip of the needle being advanced into the posterior wall or, less often, pulled from the vein whilst the syringe is being attached or removed. Rescan and reposition the needle.
  (b) The needle angle may be too steep, leading to a sharp angulation of the wire as it enters

the vein. The needle should be flattened towards the skin.
  (c) The lower part of the internal jugular vein or the innominate vein is stenosed or occluded distally. This can only be reli-ably confirmed by injecting contrast under screening control. Sometimes rotating or manipulating the wire will allow it to pass.

(2) Blood cannot be aspirated.
  (a) This is usually due to the needle tip not being in the vein. The vein wall may have been "tented" and not punctured.
  (b) Rarely there is thrombus within the needle. This can occur with repeated access attempts.

(3) The carotid artery has been punctured.
  (a) Yes. This does occasionally occur and is not uncommon with inexperienced oper-ators. (See point 1 of technique.) The needle should be withdrawn and firm pres-sure placed over the puncture for at least 5 mins. This leads to problems when the patient's clotting is prolonged by taking anticoagulants or by disease. The puncture site should be observed for at least one hour for hematoma formation, which can develop very suddenly, leading to airway obstruction.

Where can ultrasound be particularly helpful?

(1) Anticipated failure of landmark technique.
(2) Occluded jugular veins. Ultrasound can be used to find large alternative "collateral" ves-sels that may not be palpable. Veins such as the anterior jugular can be used for central access, albeit with smaller catheters.
(3) Children and neonates. Everything is smaller and it is easier to pass straight through the vein.
(4) Hypovolemic patients where veins can be col-lapsed even in the Trendelenburg position.

(5) Femoral lines in the hypovolemic or obese patient when there is difficulty palpating the femoral pulse and gaining access with the landmark technique.

(6) Ultrasound can be very useful for placing any intravenous cannulae in the "nightmare venous access patient". I always enjoy being told by patients that I will not succeed. I usually only resort to ultrasound when all the usual veins have been exhausted. Then it is very easy to find a deeper vein in the forearm or the brachial vein, which can be punctured under direct ultrasound guidance.

When you should call for help

We all fail on occasion and sometimes it is through no fault of our own!

It is important to recognize when you are unable to retrieve the situation and call for further help, perhaps from an interventional radiologist.

(1) Patients with abnormal coagulation such that inadvertent arterial puncture would be very dangerous. Using a micropuncture set can minimize the risk.

(2) If the guide wire will not advance then suspect either central stenosis or an occlusion. Further imaging will be needed.

(3) If a subsequent CXR shows the line to be misplaced into the azygous vein or even across the midline into the contralateral jugular vein. These lines can often be repositioned in the interventional suite.

(4) Patients with known previous central venous access problems, such as patients on long-term dialysis with central venous stenosis. A magnetic resonance venogram (MRV) or contrast venogram prior to an access attempt can be helpful.

(5) Patients with occluded jugular veins may have patent brachiocephalic veins/SVC. In this case it is sometimes possible for an interventional radiologist to puncture directly onto the SVC with a fine needle following placing a guidewire in the SVC stump from the groin. This tract can then be dilated and a line placed.

(6) Lines can also be placed directly onto the IVC via a lumbar approach and into the hepatic veins. These are usually routes of last resort.

Conclusion

Central venous access is usually straightforward. The use of ultrasound eliminates some of the uncertainties and undoubtedly makes the procedure safer. However, its use does require some training. There are many courses available aimed specifically at its use in venous access. If you attempt ultrasound-guided central venous access without training you will probably find an increased complication rate. This is due to lack of awareness of the common pitfalls and perhaps a degree of overconfidence.

The equipment available is reasonably priced and, like all electronics, is becoming cheaper almost by the day. It is simple to use and convenient, making its use on ITU, in anesthetic rooms and on the wards easy. It is vital to be aware of your own limitations (as in any procedure) and know when to ask for help from a more experienced colleague or interventional radiologist.

Remember that NICE does not insist on its use, but does recommend it. There is a wealth of evidence supporting its use and in the future it may become difficult to defend your use of the landmark method in the face of a serious complication.

The following quote from David Scott's *BJA* editorial sums things up [8]:

In the country of the blind, the one-eyed man is king. (Erasmus, 1466–1536).

REFERENCES

1. Elliot TSJ, Faroqui MH, Armstrong RF, Hanson GC. Guidelines for good practice in central venous catheterization. *Journal of Hospital Infection* 1994;28:163–76.

2. Reid CW. Unintentional transthoracic pulmonary artery cannulation: a complication of central line insertion. *Anesthesiology* 1995; 82:1526–8.

3. Miyamoto Y. Cervical puncture in a neonate: a rare complication of internal jugular veinpuncture. *Anesthesiology* 1996;84:1239–42.

4. National Institute for Clinical Excellence. Guidance on the use of ultrasound locating devices for placing central venous catheters. NICE technology appraisal No. 49. London, NICE, 2002.

5. Gualtieri E, Deppe SA, Sipperly ME, Thompson DR. Subclavian venous catheterization – greater success rate for less experienced operators using ultrasound guidance. *Critical Care Medicine* 1995;23:692–7.

6. Hilty WM, Hudson PA, Levitt MA, Hall JB. Real-time ultrasound-guided femoral vein catheterization during cardiopulmonary resuscitation . . . including commentary by Heller M. *Annals of Emergency Medicine* 1997;29(3):331–7.

7. Caridi JG, Hawkins IF Jr, Wiechmann BN, Pevarski DJ, Tonkin JC. Sonographic guidance when using the right internal jugular vein for central vein access. *American Journal of Radiology* 1998;171:1259–63.

8. Scott DHT. Editorial 2. It's NICE to see in the dark. *British Journal of Anaesthesia* 1999;82:820–1.

Chapter 3

Diagnostic echocardiography

TOM INGRAM

An introduction to echocardiography

It is the ability of echocardiography to assess the physiological function of the heart which is where it is of most use in anesthesiology. Echo allows a prediction of how the body's cardiovascular system will react to the stresses placed upon it by major surgery and pharmacotherapy. It is particularly suited to the analysis of valvular and ventricular function, which together account for the majority of reasons for referral. It is also useful in pericardial disease, especially pericardial effusions, and in the detection of cardiac shunts. A cause behind an arrhythmia may be identified, such as a ventricular wall scar as a nidus for ventricular tachycardia, or an enlarged left atrium causing atrial fibrillation. Where standard echocardiography is of less use is in the assessment of threatened coronary disease. Established cardiac damage will be apparent as a region of abnormal myocardial wall movement, which can be roughly approximated to the corresponding coronary arterial territory. However, other investigative tools such as exercise tolerance testing, stress echocardiography, coronary angiography or, in the future, cardiac magnetic resonance imaging are necessary to detect labile ischemic myocardium.

Echo is a powerful tool, but in order to gain the most from a study it is important not to rely upon individual values in isolation. Instead, a balanced conclusion should be reached through assessment of the heart's structural appearance in a variety of views and using different echo modalities. For example, a jet of mitral regurgitation may appear to be severe with color flow Doppler imaging, but in the chronic setting in the absence of significant ventricular or atrial dilatation it is unlikely to be so.

Standard echo windows

Some figures are printed in the text to aid understanding. All the figures are in the related Chapter 3 Power-Point file starting with The use of ultrasound in diagnostic cardiology (Intro).

Echocardiography is performed with the subject lying in the left lateral position, allowing gravity to press the heart against the chest wall (Figure 3.1, on DVD). The left hand is placed above the head to both ensure that the precordium is free from obstruction and expand the intercostal spaces. It is possible to be positioned either to the subject's left with the echo probe in your left hand, or to their right with your right arm holding the probe and looping over their torso (Figure 3.2). Finally, identify the echo probe's orientation marker, which is along one of its shorter sides (Figure 3.3).

The images produced when the heart is transected in different planes are known as echo *windows*.

Ultrasound in Anesthetic Practice, ed. Graham Arthurs and Barry Nicholls. Published by Cambridge University Press.
© Cambridge University Press 2009.

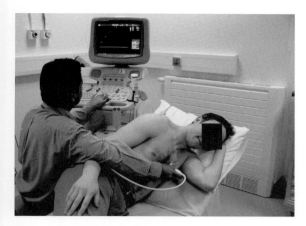

Figure 3.2 Position of echo-operator.

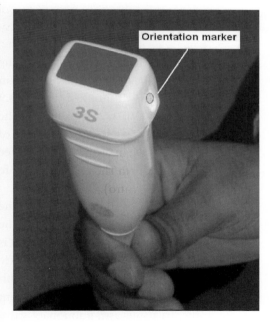

Figure 3.3 Echo machine and probe.
(Note orientation marker to the right of the probe)

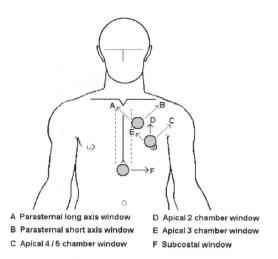

A Parasternal long axis window   D Apical 2 chamber window
B Parasternal short axis window   E Apical 3 chamber window
C Apical 4 / 5 chamber window   F Subcostal window

Figure 3.4 Probe position for six classic windows.

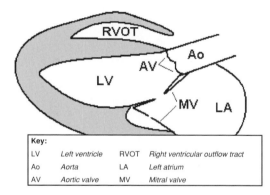

Key:			
LV	Left ventricle	RVOT	Right ventricular outflow tract
Ao	Aorta	LA	Left atrium
AV	Aortic valve	MV	Mitral valve

Figure 3.5 Parasternal long axis window.

There are two main sites from which the heart is examined, each giving rise to a number of windows according to the orientation of the probe (Figure 3.4). At the top of the heart, between the 3rd and 4th ribs at the left sternal edge, lie the parasternal long and short axis windows. At the apex of the heart are the apical *two*, *three* (*long axis*), *four* and *five*

chamber windows. Just below the xiphisternum is the *subcostal* window. These surface anatomy landmarks for each window should be taken as a rough guide, but due to anatomical variance it is better to familiarize oneself with the screen image desired and adjust the probe until this can be found. For example, the heart of a patient with hyper-expanded lungs will be pulled downwards and rotated thus moving all windows infero-medially.

(1) The parasternal long axis.

A standard echocardiogram begins with this window. The view is a longitudinal cut though the top of the heart to its base (Figure 3.5). It allows a brief overview of the left ventricle, the

25

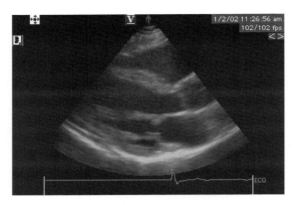

Figure 3.6   Parasternal long axis window. (normal)

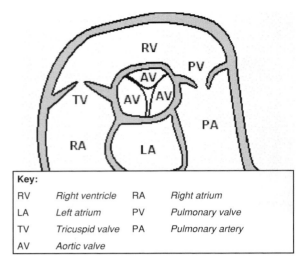

Key:			
RV	*Right ventricle*	RA	*Right atrium*
LA	*Left atrium*	PV	*Pulmonary valve*
TV	*Tricuspid valve*	PA	*Pulmonary artery*
AV	*Aortic valve*		

Figure 3.11   Parasternal short axis window, aortic valve level.

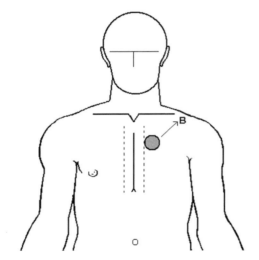

Figure 3.8   Position of probe for parasternal short axis window.

right ventricular outflow tract, the mitral and the aortic valves (Figure 3.6).

Place the probe to the left sternal edge in the space between the 3rd and 4th ribs, with the orientation marker directed towards the right shoulder (Figures 3.7, on DVD, and 3.8). If the window proves difficult to obtain, the probe should be gently tilted upwards or downwards, and then twisted. If that fails, try moving up or down a rib space.

(2) The parasternal short axis windows.

Rotate the probe from the parasternal long axis position 90° clockwise, so the orientation marker now faces the left shoulder (Figures 3.9 and 3.10, both on DVD). Angulations of the probe up and down, tilting with the axis of the orientation marker, open the standard three windows available from this position. These are the:

(a) *Aortic valve window.* This is a view of the three aortic valve leaflets *en face*, with the right heart surrounding them. To the left is the right atrium; above the right ventricle and to the right is the main trunk of the pulmonary artery (Figure 3.11). Assessment of aortic, tricuspid and pulmonary valve function is possible from this echo image (Figure 3.12).

(b) *Mitral valve window.* This is a view of the two leaflets of the mitral valve *en face*, with the body of the right ventricle to the left of the image (Figure 3.13). This view is useful for examining the opening pattern of the mitral valve which classically has been said to resemble that of a fish's mouth opening (Figure 3.14).

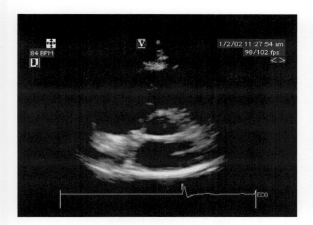

Figure 3.12 Parasternal short axis window, aortic valve level.

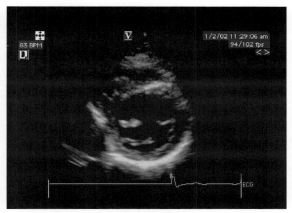

Figure 3.14 Parasternal short axis window, mitral valve level.

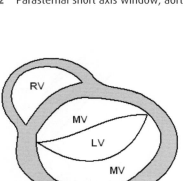

Key:			
RV	Right ventricle	LV	Left ventricle
MV	Mitral valve		

Figure 3.13 Parasternal short axis window, mitral valve level.

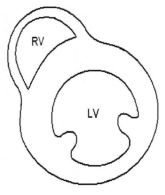

Figure 3.15 Parasternal short axis window, mitral valve apparatus level.

(c) *Mitral valve apparatus window.* This view is of the papillary muscles and chordae which support the two leaflets of the mitral valve (Figure 3.15). It allows assessment of the integrity of these structures, as well as both left and right ventricular function and dimensions (Figure 3.16, on DVD).

(3) The apical 4, 5, 2 and 3 (long axis) chamber windows.

Place the probe at the apex of the heart, either by feeling for the apex beat or locating the 6th intercostal space in the mid-clavicular line (Figures 3.17 and 3.18, both on DVD). With the orientation marker directed to the left shoulder the *apical 4-chamber* window will come into view (Figure 3.19). This is a cut from the apex of the heart across all of its four major chambers, (the left and right atria and ventricles). From this view, an assessment of these chambers and the valves separating them can be made (Figure 3.20). By tilting the probe slightly caudally the ascending aorta can be brought into view. This is the *apical 5-chamber* window (Figures 3.21 and 3.22, on DVD).

In the same position, rotate the probe 60° anti-clockwise to open up the *apical two chamber*

27

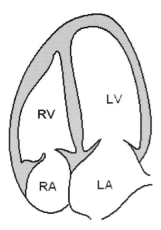

Figure 3.19   Apical 4 chamber window.

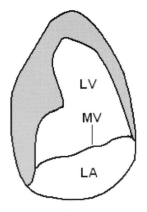

Figure 3.23   Apical 2 chamber window.

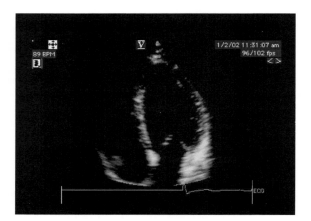

Figure 3.20   Apical 4 chamber window.

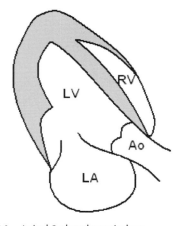

Figure 3.24   Apical 3 chamber window.

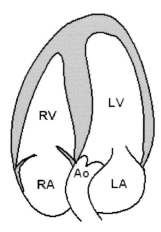

Figure 3.21   Apical 5 chamber window.

window (Figures 3.23 and 3.25, on DVD). Often the lateral wall of the left ventricle is not visible, but it can be brought into view by asking the subject to take a small breath in. By rotating the probe a further 30° anticlockwise, so that the orientation marker points towards the right shoulder, the *apical 3-chamber* (*long axis*) window is seen (Figures 3.24 and 3.26, on DVD).

These two windows are useful for assessing the motion patterns of different walls of the left ventricle, as well as providing an alternative angle from which a jet of mitral or aortic regurgitation can be assessed.

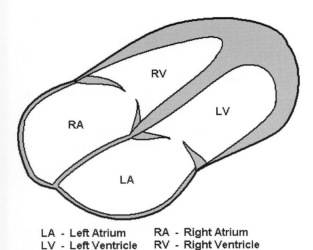

LA - Left Atrium   RA - Right Atrium
LV - Left Ventricle   RV - Right Ventricle

Figure 3.29 Subcostal window.

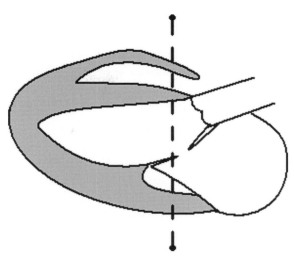

Figure 3.31 M-mode cursor alignment across the left and right ventricles in the parasternal long axis.

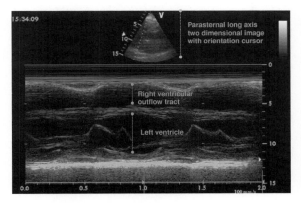

Figure 3.32 M-mode image of the left ventricle at the level of the mitral valve leaflet tips.

(4) The subcostal window.

Place the probe just below the xiphisternum in the epigastrium to obtain the *subcostal* echo window (Figures 3.27 and 3.28, both on DVD). This view is an oblique cut of the four major heart chambers (Figures 3.29 and 3.30, on DVD). The subcostal window is useful for examining right ventricular size and function and the atrial septum.

To obtain the above windows, it is necessary to adjust the echo machine settings. In particular, the depth (distance of tissue penetration) and gain (contrast) of the image will need to be optimized in each view.

Different echo modalities

Echo windows are initially examined in two-dimensional ultrasound. Heart structure and function can be further assessed in these same windows by applying the different echo modalities of: M-mode imaging (motion mode) and Doppler waveform imaging (color or pulsed/continuous).

M-mode (motion mode) imaging

This was the first form of echocardiography developed. A single ultrasound beam is transmitted and its reflection listened for along a single line of the two-dimensional window's imaging sweep. The resultant signal trace is then mapped across the screen over time. The role of M-mode imaging is to show the pattern of movement of cardiac structures, and provide a still picture for their measurement. For instance, an M-mode image taken across the left ventricle in the parasternal long axis window will show the systolic and then diastolic motion of both anterior and posterior left ventricular walls (Figures 3.31 and 3.32). The caveat of this modality is that any measurements taken are entirely dependent on the original cut made. An oblique M-mode image will overestimate a cavity's dimensions markedly. For this reason, any measurements taken should never be used in isolation to make a clinical decision.

Doppler waveform imaging

Christian Andreas Doppler, an Austrian physicist, has given his name to the Doppler Effect. He described a phenomenon affecting light waves. He observed that the colors emitted by the stars change depending on whether the star is moving towards or away from the observer. This is due to the change in frequency of the radiation: higher if the two are moving towards or a lower frequency if moving apart from each other.

He observed the same phenomenon with sound waves: that a sound emitted from a moving object is different when the object is moving towards the receiver than when it is moving away from the receiver. The sound is of a higher frequency (pitch) when the object moves towards the observer and a lower frequency when moving away.

The same principle is used in echocardiography: blood flow towards an echo probe produces an ultrasound reflection of a greater frequency than it was originally emitted with (a *shift* in frequency), and vice versa. The Doppler shift principle has three major uses in echo.

PULSED WAVE DOPPLER IMAGING

A short pulse of ultrasound is emitted, which is then listened for once a set period of time has elapsed. As the speed of sound is constant through the heart, the period of time between these two events determines the depth at which the velocity of blood is analyzed. Whilst this method allows precise evaluation of flow at a particular point in the heart, the main drawback is that high velocity jets of blood suffer a problem known as *"aliasing"*. This is when the minimum repeat rate over which the signal must be

sampled is too quick and the frequency shift measured is thus inaccurate. The signal therefore loops over one end of the screen to the other (Figure 3.33, on DVD).

Pulsed wave Doppler imaging can be used to analyze blood flow across the mitral valve, and in so doing calculate the mitral valve orifice area (Figure 3.34, on DVD). It is also used in the calculation of cardiac output and shunts.

COLOR FLOW DOPPLER

Improvement in computer processing speeds has meant that several points across an imaging arc can have their pulsed wave Doppler shift frequency measured simultaneously. This allows a two-dimensional real-time representation of cardiac hemodynamics, which is displayed in different colors. By convention, red signifies flow towards the transducer and blue flow away from it (BART – Blue Away Red Towards).

Color flow Doppler imaging is used to assess jets of valvular regurgitation and shunts between cardiac chambers (Figure 3.35, on DVD). As with pulsed wave Doppler imaging, aliasing occurs and high-velocity jets of blood traveling in either direction are displayed in white or green. It is important to emphasize that aliasing indicates a high velocity of a single point of flow and not overall flow volume. It therefore represents a high pressure difference between two chambers, and is not in itself a marker of the severity of a leak.

CONTINUOUS WAVE DOPPLER

This is a process similar to pulsed wave Doppler imaging. The probe both transmits ultrasound and listens for the reflections produced simultaneously. The issue of a minimum repeat rate is thus avoided and no aliasing at higher velocities occurs. However, the ability to locate blood velocity at a specific position is lost. This is because flow velocity at all points along the chosen line of imaging are assessed and then averaged to a single reading. This is then displayed over time in a spectral flow image.

Continuous wave Doppler imaging is used to assess high-velocity blood flow as occurs with aortic stenosis (Figure 3.36, on DVD).

Some normal echo variants

Figure references relate to Normal variants Power-Point file on the DVD: The use of ultrasound in diagnostic cardiology normal variants.

(1) Trivial mitral regurgitation (Figure 3.v.1).

(2) Minor aortic valve tip thickening and calcification without an associated flow gradient (Figure 3.v.2). This often causes a systolic murmur and is sometimes referred to as aortic sclerosis. It is particularly common in the elderly.

(3) Sub-aortic septal bulge to the septum of the left ventricle (Figure 3.v.3). This is due to fibrosis of myocardium in the elderly.

(4) Moderator band in the right ventricular apex. This is an echogenic band of tissue which contains conduction tract material from the His–Purkinje system.

Case 1. Assessing left ventricular function

PowerPoint file: The use of ultrasound in diagnostic cardiology (CASE 1).

Scenario

A 65-year-old man attends a pre-operative assessment clinic for an inguinal hernia repair. He had a myocardial infarction 10 years previously and has not been troubled by angina since then. Over recent months, he has noticed that he is unable to walk his granddaughter the quarter mile it is to her local school due to a shortage of breath. He is also waking breathless at night twice a week.

On examination he has a pulse of 96 beats per minute, which is regular, and blood pressure of 110/70 mmHg. Precordial auscultation reveals a third heart sound but no murmurs. He has coarse inspiratory crackles to the mid-zones of his chest bilaterally, and pitting oedema up to his thighs. The electrocardiogram (ECG) shows a left bundle branch block. You wish to perform echocardiography.

Discussion

The main role of echo in this gentleman is to assess his left ventricular systolic function. In particular echo can identify specific regional wall motion abnormalities, corresponding to the territory of a previous myocardial infarction. This abnormal motion is categorized as: *hypokinetic* (reduced), *akinetic* (absent) or *dyskinetic* (paradoxical to that expected). Scarring (thinning) and aneurysms of the ventricular walls can also be seen. There is no one test for assessing left ventricular function at echo. Rather a combination of both two-dimensional and M-mode imaging in different windows is used to gain an overall impression (Table 3.1).

Initial assessment of left ventricular systolic function should be by quick visual *"eyeballing"* in the major windows. In the parasternal long axis window the interventricular septum (IVS) is above and the left ventricular posterior wall (LVPW) is below (Figures 3.1.1, on DVD, and 3.1.2). The apex is not seen in this window. Examine the ventricular wall dimensions; they will be thickened with left ventricular hypertrophy or thin with ischemic scarring. Also look at each wall's motion relative to other

Table 3.1 Normal values of the left ventricle (for adults)

Wall thickness	(diastole)	6–12 mm
	(systole)	9–18 mm
LVEDD		35–36 mm
LVESD		20–56 mm
Ejection fraction	50–85%	

LVEDD = Left Ventricular End Diastolic Diameter
LVESD = Left Ventricular End Systolic Diameter

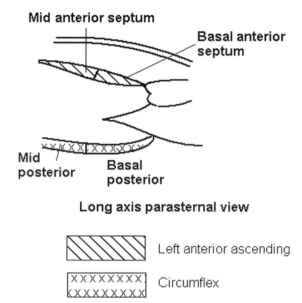

Long axis parasternal view

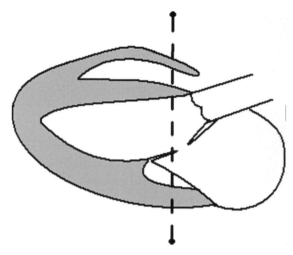

Figure 3.1.3 M-mode cursor alignment across the left and right ventricles in the parasternal long axis.

Figure 3.1.2 Parasternal long axis view. Arterial blood supply.

parts of the ventricle; if function is poor it can be regional or global to the whole ventricle. The same process should be repeated in the parasternal short axis window (mitral valve apparatus level) and apical 4 and 2 chamber windows. This gives an assessment of the whole left ventricle (Figure 3.1.2).

Next, line up the cursor across the body of the left ventricle in the parasternal long axis window, just at the level of the mitral valve leaflet tips, and switch to M-mode (Figures 3.1.3 and 3.1.4). The image produced shows how the IVS and LVPW move during the cardiac cycle, and with calculation a crude estimate of the left ventricular ejection fraction can be made.

On this M-mode image use the calliper tool to measure the left ventricular end systolic diameter (LVESD). This should be from the endocardium of the IVS to the endocardium of the LVPW at the point where there is the minimum gap between two, which roughly coincides with the *t wave* of the ECG. Care should be taken as it is easy to confuse the mitral valve apparatus with the endocardium. The left ventricular end diastolic diameter

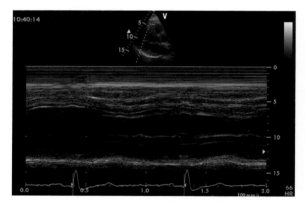

Figure 3.1.4 M-mode image across the left ventricle.

(LVEDD) should then be measured. This is similar from endocardium to endocardium of the ventricle, but at the point of its maximum diameter, which coincides with the *R wave* of the ECG. From these figures the left ventricular ejection fraction can be calculated:

Ejection fraction (*normal* 50−85%)
$$= \frac{(LVEDD)^3 - (LVESD)^3}{(LVEDD)^3} \times 100\%$$

(Note: this method of calculating the ejection fraction assumes the ventricle to be an ellipse and generally give an overestimated result.) Ventricular wall

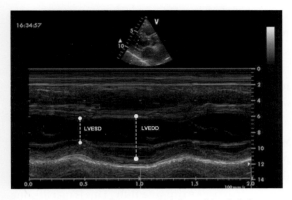

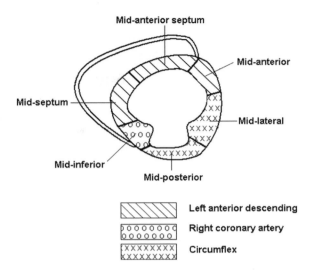

Figure 3.1.6   M-mode imaging of the subject's left ventricle – septal wall hypokinesia.

Figure 3.1.8   Parasternal short axis window.

thickness can also be measured on this M-mode image, in both diastole (normal 6–12 mm) and systole (normal 9–18 mm).

The echo of this gentleman shows him to have a hypokinetic (virtually akinetic) septal wall in the parasternal long axis window (Figures 3.1.5 and 3.1.1 normal, both on DVD). An M-mode image across the left ventricle in this window reveals that the IVS does not move significantly during the cardiac cycle, but the LVPW does (Figures 3.1.6 and 3.1.4 normal, on DVD). His estimated ejection frac-

tion is a generous 40–50%. The parasternal short axis (Figures 3.1.7, on DVD, 3.1.8 and 3.1.9 normal, on DVD) and apical 4-chamber (Figures 3.1.10, on DVD, 3.1.11 and 3.1.12 normal, on DVD) windows also display antero-septal hypokinesia.

This gentleman's echo study is consistent with a previous myocardial infarction to the left coronary circulation, most probably in the LAD territory. He

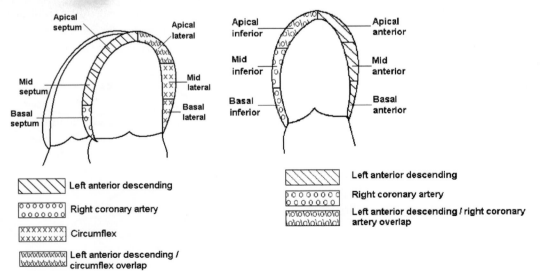

Figure 3.1.11   Apical 4-chamber view. Arterial blood supply. Apical 2-chamber view. Arterial blood supply. Figures show left ventricle wall with its associated arterial blood supply territories.

has moderate left ventricular impairment. Anesthesia would be risky, given his clinical decompensated cardiac state, and surgery should be postponed until this is optimized.

Further examples

For comparison, three extra sets of echo images are included. The first is of an athlete's heart; note the strong movement of all regions of the ventricle (Figures 3.1.13 and 3.1.14, both on DVD). The second is of a septal aneurysm, occurring post myocardial infarction (Figures 3.1.15 and 3.1.16, both on DVD). The third set of images shows a case of dilated cardiomyopathy, with global hypokinesia to left ventricular wall motion (Figure 3.1.18, on DVD). The apical 4-chamber window of this patient reveals an associated, functional, mitral regurgitation due to dilatation of the mitral valve annulus (Figure 3.1.19, on DVD).

Case 2. Assessing mitral regurgitation

PowerPoint file: The use of ultrasound in diagnostic cardiology (CASE 2).

Scenario

A 78-year-old lady is admitted with a fractured neck of femur following slipping on ice whilst out shopping. She had a myocardial infarction 2 years ago, from which she made a good recovery, and has no other past medical history of note.

On examination her pulse is 80 beats per minutes and regular. Her blood pressure is 160/90 mmHg. Precordial auscultation reveals a harsh pan-systolic murmur which radiates to the left axilla. On listening to her chest, she has bi-basal crackles. Venous pressure is not raised and there is no peripheral oedema. You wish to perform echocardiography.

Discussion

The clinical diagnosis in this case is mitral regurgitation. Echo will give useful information as to the origin and severity of this valvular lesion, how the left ventricle has been affected, and whether an alternative diagnosis is more likely (e.g. aortic stenosis or a ventricular septal defect). Mitral regurgitation can be caused by a number of reasons, relating to damage to the different structures necessary for valvular integrity (Figure 3.2.1). The leaflets can be affected, either by direct destruction, as is the case with endocarditis, degenerative changes, or their prolapse during systole. The annulus surrounding the leaflets may be dilated, resulting in an inability of the valve cusps to oppose fully. This is usually due to dilatation of the left ventricle. Mitral regurgitation can also be secondary to rupture of a papillary muscle or chordae, which are collectively known as the mitral valve apparatus. The exact cause of regurgitation is of particular importance if surgery is being considered. This is because repair to a damaged valve leaflet may be more appropriate than whole valve replacement, or a ring annuloplasty procedure may be used to correct dilatation of the mitral annulus.

To examine for mitral regurgitation on echo, the first window used is the parasternal long axis. This view allows a quick assessment of valvular and ventricular structure and function. The natural pathophysiology of chronic mitral regurgitation is towards left ventricular *dilatation* with hyperdynamic motion due to volume overload, but not

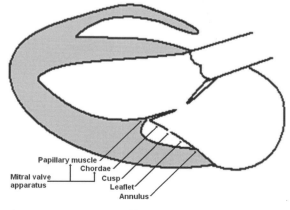

Figure 3.2.1 Parasternal long axis view showing the structures constituting the Mitral valve.

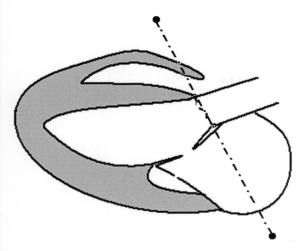

Figure 3.2.2 Parasternal long axis window – position of cursor alignment for M-mode imaging of the aortic valve and left atrium.

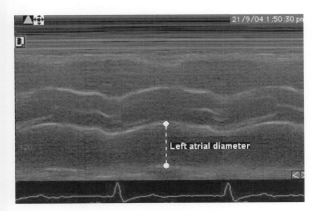

Figure 3.2.3 M-mode imaging across the aortic valve and left atrium (normal).

hypertrophy. The methods for assessing ventricular cavity and wall sizes are outlined in Case 1. Valvular motion should also be examined for prolapse of either leaflet into the left atrium during systole or an associated mitral stenosis (see Case 5).

Next, align the cursor with the aortic valve tips and switch to M-mode imaging (Figures 3.2.2 and 3.2.3). In this view, use the calliper tool to measure the maximum diameter of the left atrium (nor-

mal 20–45 mm). Mitral regurgitation causes volume overload of the left atrium, and consequently over time it will dilate. This structural change is a significant substrate for atrial fibrillation.

Now apply color flow Doppler imaging to the parasternal long axis window, focusing on the mitral valve and left atrium. Mitral regurgitation appears as a blue (or even white/green if flow velocity is high and *aliased*) jet into the left atrium during ventricular systole. Often the jet will originate from the center of the valve, particularly if it is due to mitral annular dilatation. It can be quite eccentric (i.e. at an acute angle to the valve), particularly if the cause is a mitral leaflet prolapse.

To assess the severity of regurgitation, the volume of blood which is traveling from the ventricle back into the atrium needs to be quantified. This volume is proportional to the size of the base of the regurgitant jet, whether recruitment of the jet begins within the left ventricle and the volume of the left atrium that it fills. (N.B. this last marker will underestimate the jet's severity if the left atrium is dilated.) The jet is best visualized in the apical windows by gently tilting the probe up and down until its maximum dimensions have been found.

Mitral regurgitation is graded as: trivial, mild, moderate or severe. Trivial regurgitation has a narrow base, extends less than 1 cm into the atrium and does not last for the whole of systole. Mild regurgitation is similar, but lasts for the whole of systole and can extend up to half way into the atrium. In moderate regurgitation the jet reaches the back of the atrium and is of a broader base. Much aliasing will occur, and a blue arc extends from the ventricular side of the valve as recruitment of blood into the jet takes place from within the ventricle. Severe regurgitation can fill the whole of the atrium.

(N.B. If tachycardia renders color flow Doppler imaging difficult to interpret in real time, then the image should be frozen and the cardiac cycle slowly rewound through.)

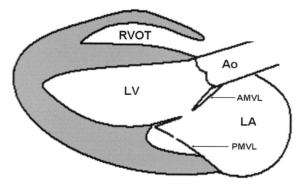

Figure 3.2.5 Parasternal long axis window with both of the mitral valve leaflets illustrated.

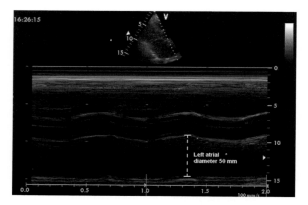

Figure 3.2.9 M-mode imaging across the subject's aortic valve and left atrium.

The echo windows of the lady in this case demonstrate that she has a prolapse of her posterior mitral valve leaflet (PMVL) (Figures 3.2.4, on DVD, 3.2.5 and 3.2.6 normal, on DVD). This is causing an eccentric jet of mitral regurgitation that is directed anteriorly towards the aortic root (Figures 3.2.7 and 3.2.8 normal, both on DVD). An M-mode image taken across her left atrium shows it to be dilated; however, this value should be used with caution, as the cut is clearly oblique (Figure 3.2.9).

The parasternal short axis window at the level of the mitral valve apparatus further explains the underlying pathology behind this lady's mitral regurgitation. The inferior wall of the left ventricle

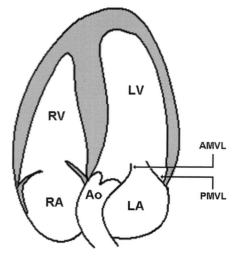

Figure 3.2.14 Apical 5-chamber window with both of the mitral valve leaflets illustrated.

is hypokinetic, thin and aneurismal (Figures 3.2.10, 3.2.11 and 3.2.12 normal, all on DVD). This is the result of a previous inferior myocardial infarction. The papillary muscle that stabilizes the posterior mitral valve leaflet receives an exclusive blood supply from the right coronary artery, as opposed to the anterior papillary muscle which has a dual blood supply from both the right and left coronary beds. This lady has suffered an ischemic rupture of her posterior papillary muscle.

The severity of this lady's mitral regurgitation can be quantified in her apical 4/5 chamber window. The prolapsed PMVL is clearer in this view. Also note the large size of the left atrium and hyperdynamic motion of the dilated left ventricle (Figures 3.2.13, on DVD, 3.2.14 and 3.2.15 normal, on DVD). These features suggest that the regurgitation is at least moderate. Color flow Doppler imaging in the apical 5 chamber window show that the regurgitant jet has a broad base. It is reflected off the aortic wall of the atrium and extends back to fill nearly the whole of this cavity. This is therefore severe mitral regurgitation (Figures 3.2.16 and 3.2.17 normal, both on DVD).

MILD

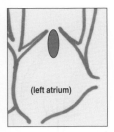

(left atrium)

Small base to jet

Extends partially into the LA

Normal LA / LV dimensions

SEVERE

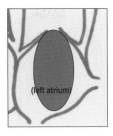

(left atrium)

Broad base to jet

Fills much of the LA

Dilated   LA / LV

Figure 3.2.22   Summary of mild vs. severe mitral regurgitation.

Further examples

Figures 3.2.18a and 3.2.18b (on DVD) illustrate how easy it is to underestimate the severity of mitral regurgitation if several different windows are not looked at in its assessment. Figures 3.2.19 and 3.2.20 (on DVD) are of mild mitral regurgitation. Figures 3.2.21a and 3.2.21b (on DVD) show an anterior mitral valve leaflet prolapse, with bowing of this leaflet into the atrium and a posterior eccentric jet of mild mitral regurgitation. Figure 3.2.22 is a summary of the differentiating features between mild and severe mitral regurgitation.

Case 3. Assessing aortic stenosis

PowerPoint file: The use of ultrasound in diagnostic cardiology (CASE 3).

Scenario

A 63-year-old keen gardener has severe osteoarthritis of his left knee and is awaiting a total knee replacement. At pre-operative assessment, he tells you that he has been progressively becoming more short of breath on exertion for the last 8 months. However, he has still been able to work and puts his symptoms down to "old age". He also tells you

that 7 weeks ago he had an episode of loss of consciousness without warning whilst gardening.

On examination he has a pulse of 70 beats per minute, which is regular, and a blood pressure of 170/110 mmHg. Heart auscultation reveals a soft ESM radiating to both carotid arteries, and a soft second heart sound. His apex beat is forceful but not displaced. Chest examination is unremarkable, venous pressure is not elevated, and no peripheral oedema is present. ECG shows large voltage complexes across the chest leads, consistent with left ventricular hypertrophy. You wish to perform echocardiography.

Discussion

The clinical diagnosis here is that of aortic stenosis. This is usually the result of degenerative calcification of the aortic valve, although rheumatic fever and a congenitally bicuspid valve may accelerate this process. Echo is useful to ascertain the severity of any aortic valve orifice narrowing, or to identify an alternative diagnosis such as left ventricular outflow tract obstruction with hypertrophic obstructive cardiomyopathy. Narrowing of the aortic valve orifice causes an increase in the workload of the left ventricle, but without significant volume overload. The natural progression of aortic stenosis therefore is towards global left ventricular hypertrophy, with dilatation of the ventricle only occurring as a late feature of decompensated disease.

Assessment of aortic stenosis should begin in the parasternal long axis window (Figure 3.3.1, on DVD). This window provides a quick view of both the aortic valve and the left ventricle. Using the methods outlined in Case 1, the left ventricular cavity and wall sizes can be measured and an ejection fraction estimated. Now concentrate on the aortic valve and how well the leaflets separate during systole. In valvular stenosis, the leaflets may be stiff and appear bright due to calcification. With a severely calcified, stenosed, valve the movements of individual leaflets will not be distinguishable, and the

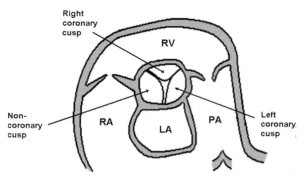

Figure 3.3.4 Parasternal short axis window: aortic valve level illustrating the different cusps of the aortic valve. RV, right ventricle; PA, pulmonary artery; RA, right atrium; LA, left atrium.

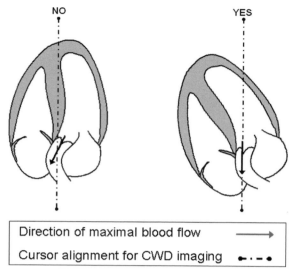

| Direction of maximal blood flow | → |
| Cursor alignment for CWD imaging | ●–·–● |

Figure 3.3.5 Alignment of the cursor for CWD imaging of aortic blood flow.

valve will appear as a piece of "chalk" throwing an acoustic shadow into the left atrium.

Stay in the parasternal long axis window and line up the cursor across the aortic valve for an M-mode image (Figures 3.3.2 and 3.3.3, both on DVD). This picture shows a "window" of the valve opening during systole, which is narrower if any stenosis is present. In severe stenosis, the whole window is obscured with echo shadows. The diameter of the aortic root is also measured in this view (normal 20–35 mm). This is of particular importance if aortic valve surgery is being contemplated, as dilatation may necessitate replacement of both the aortic valve and root.

Now change to the parasternal short axis window at the level of the aortic valve (Figure 3.3.4). This *en face* view of the valve is useful for assessing its structure and orifice size. The usual Y-shape produced by the valve's three cusps may be distorted if stenosis is present. This can be due to a congenitally bicuspid valve, or fusion of the leaflets together at their free edges.

The best window for quantifying the severity of aortic stenosis is the apical 5 chamber. Align the probe so that the aortic valve and left ventricular outflow tract are perpendicular to the apex of the image sweep (Figure 3.3.5). This alignment is crucial, as any obliqueness to the direction of max-

imal blood flow across the aortic valve will cause an underestimation of the pressure drop across it. Once the optimum window has been found, line up the cursor across the aortic valve and switch to continuous wave Doppler imaging. The sound of blood flowing across the valve during systole is heard, which should be crisp and loud. The resulting trace produced demonstrates how the velocity of blood flow across the aortic valve varies in real time (Figure 3.3.6, on DVD). Freeze this image and use the calliper tool to measure the peak velocity of forwards flow across the valve. This will be below the baseline, as blood is flowing away from the probe. This peak velocity (in m/s) can then be converted to the pressure drop across the valve (in mmHg) by using the simplified Bernoulli equation:

$$\text{Pressure drop} = 4 \times (V_{\text{peak}})^2$$

At least three separate readings should be taken in both the apical 5 and 3 chamber windows. It is particularly important not to accept a single low-gradient reading if the valve appears calcified or the ventricle hypertrophied.

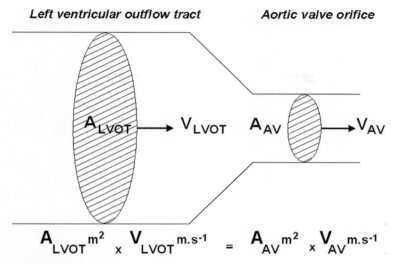

Left ventricular outflow tract   **Aortic valve orifice**

$$A_{LVOT}\,m^2 \times V_{LVOT}\,m.s^{-1} = A_{AV}\,m^2 \times V_{AV}\,m.s^{-1}$$

Figure 3.3.7   Measuring the left ventricular outflow tract diameter.

If left ventricular function is impaired in the presence of aortic stenosis, then the stroke volume will be reduced and the gradient across the valve may be underestimated using the simplified Bernoulli equation. In this situation, the cause can be either severe aortic stenosis with an associated decompensated ventricle, or milder aortic stenosis with an alternative cause of ventricular impairment (e.g. ischemic heart disease). Differentiation between these two causes is possible by using the continuity equation to calculate the cross-sectional area of the aortic valve orifice.

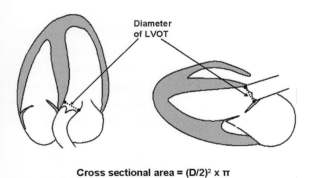

Cross sectional area = (D/2)² x π

Figure 3.3.8   Measuring the left ventricular outflow tract.

The continuity equation is based on the assumption that blood flow through the heart is in an enclosed, cylindrical system. Therefore the volume of blood, per unit time, through the aortic valve's cross-sectional area will be identical to that through a different cross-sectional area in the left ventricular outflow tract (Figure 3.3.7).

$$A_{(AV)}\,m^2 \times V_{(AV)}\,m/s^1$$
$$= A_{(LVOT)}\,m^2 \times V_{(LVOT)}\,m/s^1$$

The measurements required are from the parasternal long axis and apical 5 chamber windows. Freeze the two-dimensional image and use the callipers to measure the diameter of the cross-sectional area of the LVOT (Figures 3.3.1, 3.3.8 and 3.3.9). Assuming that this region is circular, the equation: area = Π $(D/2)^2$ can be used to calculate the cross-sectional area of the LVOT. Now line up the cursor across the aortic valve and switch to pulsed wave Doppler imaging. The cross-hairs of the PWD should be lined up at the level of the LVOT (Figures 3.3.10 and 3.3.11, both on DVD) and the peak velocity at this point measured. Now put these values, together with the peak velocity across the aortic

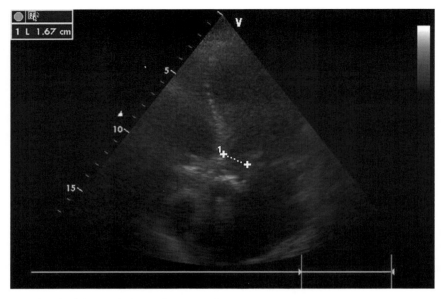

Figure 3.3.9 Measuring the left ventricular outflow tract diameter.

Table 3.2 Degrees of severity of aortic stenosis

	Peak velocity (m/s)	Peak gradient (mmHg)	Valve area (cm²)
Normal	1.0	< 10	2.5–3.5
Mild	1.0–2.0	< 20	1.5–2.5
Moderate	2.0–4.0	20–64	0.75–1.5
Severe	> 4.0	> 64	< 0.75

valve calculated earlier, into the rearranged continuity equation:

$$A_{(AV)} \; m^2 = \frac{A_{(LVOT)} \; m^2 \times V_{(LVOT)} \; m/s^1}{V_{(AV)} \; m/s^1}$$

to give the cross-sectional area of the aortic valve (Table 3.2).

The gentleman in this case has severe aortic stenosis with a hypertrophied but reasonably functioning left ventricle. The parasternal long axis window demonstrates this well, showing the aortic valve to be heavily calcified with no obvious valve leaflets identifiable (Figures 3.3.12 and 3.3.13 normal, both on DVD). An M-mode image across

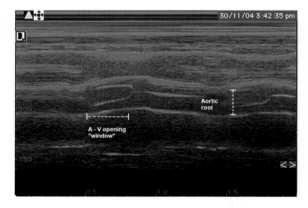

Figure 3.3.14 M-mode image across the subject's aortic valve – reduced valve opening present.

the aortic valve also shows this valvular calcification, with echo shadowing within the normal window of valve opening (Figures 3.3.14 and 3.3.15 normal, on DVD). In the parasternal short axis window, left ventricular hypertrophy can be seen (Figures 3.3.16, 3.3.17 and 3.3.18 normal, all on DVD).

In the apical 5 chamber window, the calcified and immobile aortic valve can again be seen (Figures 3.3.19, 3.3.20 and 3.3.21 normal, all on DVD). The probe is moved laterally to align the aortic valve and root with the image sweep's apex, and color flow Doppler imaging is used to show turbulence across the valve (Figure 3.3.22, on DVD). A continuous wave Doppler image is then taken across the valve (Figures 3.3.23 and 3.3.24 normal, both on DVD). The trace obtained has a peak velocity of 5 m/s and therefore the aortic valve has an estimated pressure drop of 100 mmHg across it. Surgical replacement of this valve should be considered, especially as there is a history of blackouts.

Further examples

Figure 3.3.25a (on DVD) shows an immobile lower cusp to the aortic valve in the parasternal long axis window. This can be seen to be due to fusion of the left and right coronary cusps in the parasternal short axis view (Figure 3.3.25b, on DVD). M-mode imaging of the aortic valve in the same subject demonstrates that a satisfactory opening window is still being produced by the valve (Figure 3.3.25, on DVD). This indicates that the stenosis is not severe, a fact also suggested by the well-functioning and non-hypertrophied left ventricle. Figure 3.3.26 (on DVD) is of a bicuspid aortic valve (Figure 3.3.27 normal, on DVD). Figures 3.3.28a, 3.3.28b and 3.3.28c (all on DVD) are different echo windows of a case of hypertrophic obstructive cardiomyopathy (HOCM).

Case 4. Assessing aortic regurgitation

PowerPoint file: The use of ultrasound in diagnostic cardiology (CASE 4).

Scenario

A 30-year-old man with ankylosing spondylosis is admitted for a cholecystectomy. He has previously only taken paracetamol for relief of intermittent lower back pain, and has no other symptoms of note.

On examination he has reduced flexion, extension and rotation of his cervical and lumbar spine. Pulse is 70 beats per minute, regular and collapsing in character. Blood pressure is 110/40 mmHg. Precordial auscultation reveals normal heart sounds with a loud early diastolic murmur which extends throughout the whole of diastole. Chest examination is unremarkable. There is no peripheral oedema present and venous pressure is not elevated. You wish to perform echocardiography.

Discussion

The clinical diagnosis here is that of aortic regurgitation. The etiology is most likely connected to his ankylosing spondylosis. This is a connective tissue disease which can cause aortic regurgitation through both alterations of the valvular integrity and by dilatation of the aortic root. Other causes of valvular aortic regurgitation include endocarditis, rheumatic heart disease, and a congenital bicuspid valve. Indeed, any stenosed valve is likely to have a degree of regurgitation associated with it, as the stiff leaflets are often as unable to oppose as they are to open. Diseases which may cause dilatation of the aortic root include aortic dissection, Marfan's disease, and hypertension.

Initial echo assessment of aortic regurgitation is from the parasternal long axis window. From here, an idea of left ventricular involvement in the disease can be made, and any specific etiological factors, such as vegetations attached to the valve, may be seen. The natural history of aortic regurgitation is towards ventricular volume overload and dilatation, without significant hypertrophy. Surgical treatment to replace a leaking aortic valve is, in part, directed by the left ventricular cavity size, and in particular the left ventricular end diastolic diameter (LVEDD). Details on how to measure this can be found in Case 1. The size of the LVEDD correlates with the incidence of sudden cardiac death. An M-mode image should also be taken across the aortic valve and the aortic root diameter measured (see Case 3).

Next switch to color flow Doppler imaging, whilst remaining in the parasternal long axis window. Aortic regurgitation can be seen as a blue jet of blood directed back into the left ventricle during early diastole. As with mitral regurgitation, the severity of regurgitation corresponds to: the size of the base of the jet, how far it extends back into the left ventricle, and for how long (during diastole) the jet lasts. Color flow Doppler imaging should also be observed in all of the apical windows, so that the maximum dimensions of any regurgitant jet can be located. Remember that, as with mitral regurgitation, a jet may be eccentric and thus difficult to locate.

Remain in the apical 5 chamber window and align the aortic valve and left ventricular outflow tract so that they are perpendicular to the image sweep's apex (Figure 3.4.1). Line up the cursor across the aortic valve and switch to continuous wave Doppler imaging. The trace produced will show the jet of regurgitating blood flow above the baseline during diastole (Figure 3.4.2).

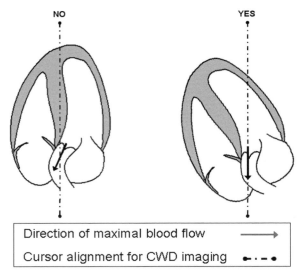

| Direction of maximal blood flow | ⟶ |
| Cursor alignment for CWD imaging | •–·–• |

Figure 3.4.1 Alignment of the CWD cursor in the apical 5 chamber window.

The degree of deceleration to the flow of this jet indicates the severity of aortic regurgitation. A flatter-topped trace suggests a small degree of back-flow without significant equalization of pressure

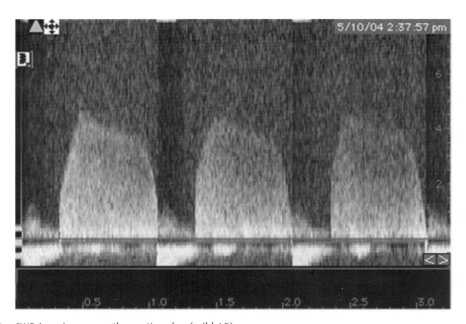

Figure 3.4.2 CWD imaging across the aortic valve (mild AR).

(a)

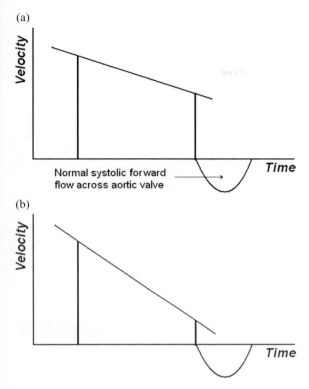

Normal systolic forward flow across aortic valve

(b)

Figures 3.4.3 CWD pattern of aortic blood flow. (a) Normal systolic forward flow across AV valve mild aortic regurgitation). (b) Severe aortic regurgitation.

between the aorta and left ventricle during diastole. However, if the jet rapidly decelerates, even reaching the baseline by the end of diastole, this suggests a sizeable orifice allowing equalization of the pressures between the aorta and ventricle (Figure 3.4.3).

This observation of the degree of deceleration in pressure change can be calculated by the echo machine using the *pressure half time* function (Figure 3.4.4). Freeze the continuous wave Doppler trace across the aortic valve and use the calliper to mark the maximum (starting) point of the trace (A) and minimum point (B). The echo machine can then calculate the time it takes for the initial pressure to drop to half the original value. A value of greater than 400 ms is considered to be mild aortic regurgitation. Care should be taken if the patient is in atrial fibrillation, as a different stroke volume will occur with each cardiac cycle, making the envelope that each jet produces different (Figure 3.4.5) (Table 3.3).

This gentleman has severe aortic regurgitation. This is indicated by his dilated but well-functioning left ventricle shown in both the parasternal long axis

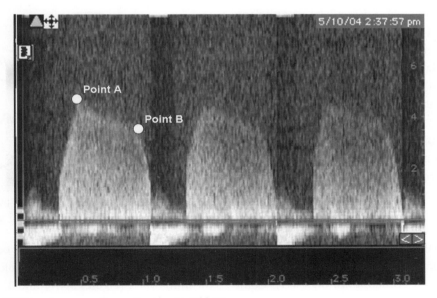

Figure 3.4.4 CWD imaging across the aortic valve in mild AR.

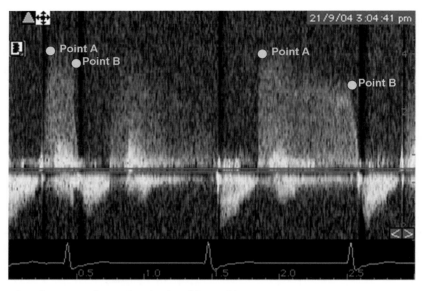

Figure 3.4.5 CWD imaging across the aortic valve in mild AR with AF.

Table 3.3 Grading the severity of aortic regurgitation

	Color flow Doppler features	Ventricular dimensions	Pressure half time of gradient between the LV and aorta
Mild	Narrow-based jet within the AV area	Normal	>400 ms
Severe	Broad-based jet extending to the ventricular apex	Dilated (LVEDD >55 mm) / poor systolic function	<400 ms

(Figures 3.4.6, on DVD, 3.4.7 and 3.4.8 normal, on DVD) and short axis windows (Figures 3.4.9, 3.4.10 and 3.4.11 normal, all on DVD). His aortic root is also mildly dilated. An M-mode image across the left ventricle, at the level of the mitral valve leaflet tips, measures the LVEDD to be enlarged at 62 mm (Figure 3.4.12). Color flow Doppler imaging in the parasternal long axis window shows a broad-based jet of eccentric aortic regurgitation (Figures 3.4.13 and 3.4.14 normal, both on DVD). The jet mixes with the normal forwards blood flow across the mitral valve during diastole, making its full extent difficult to quantify.

Switching to the apical 4/5 chamber window, the dilated ventricle can be clearly appreciated (Figures 3.4.15 and 3.4.16 normal, both on DVD). Color flow Doppler imaging in this window shows that

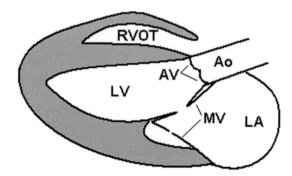

Figure 3.4.7 Parasternal long axis window. LA, left atrium; MV, mitral valve; LV, left ventricle; RVOT, right ventricle outflow tract; AO, aorta; AV, aortic valve.

the jet hugs the side of the ventricle before mixing with the normal forwards flow of blood through the mitral valve (Figures 3.4.17 and 3.4.18 normal, both on DVD). It was not possible to line up the

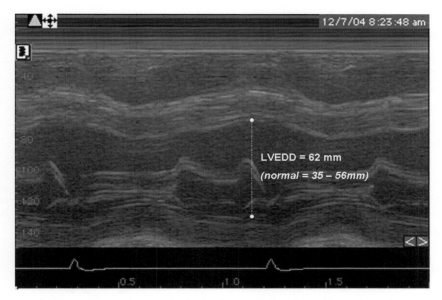

Figure 3.4.12 M-mode imaging across the mitral valve leaflet tips – dilated LV with good systolic function.

continuous wave Doppler cursor with the jet of regurgitation, given its eccentric nature. However, despite these limitations, it is possible to say that this man's aortic regurgitation is severe due to the dilatation of his left ventricle.

Even though this man is asymptomatic, he may require surgery to his aortic valve. A CT or MRI scan of his chest to assess his aortic root further would be necessary prior to surgery.

Further examples
Figure 3.4.19 (on DVD) is a case of mild aortic regurgitation, from an older patient with a mildly calcified but non-stenosed aortic valve.

Case 5. Assessing mitral stenosis
PowerPoint file: The use of ultrasound in diagnostic cardiology (CASE 5).

Scenario
A 28-year-old pregnant lady from Indonesia is having an elective cesarean section at 36 weeks due to pre-eclampsia. She had rheumatic fever as a child. She tells you that she has been getting gradually more breathless over the last 16 weeks.

On examination, she has an irregular pulse of 78 beats a minute, and a blood pressure of 140/80 mmHg. Precordial auscultation reveals a diastolic opening snap with a low pitch mid-diastolic murmur and loud first heart sound. On listening to her chest, she has bilateral crackles to the mid-zones. Her venous pressure is slightly raised and mild pedal pitting oedema is present. You wish to perform echocardiography.

Discussion
The clinical history and examination here is strongly suggestive of mitral stenosis. Mitral stenosis is almost exclusively due to rheumatic fever of childhood, a situation where cross-reactivity of streptococci cell wall antigens occurs with the heart valve tissue. The resultant inflammation causes nodular scarring to the valves, which then thicken and fibrose over time. The main areas affected are the valve commissures (where the valves join each other), cusps (free valve edges) and chordae (Figure 3.5.1, on DVD). Echo can identify these sites of fibrosis, and assess impedance to blood flow. It can also identify complications (e.g. atrial

thrombus) and rule out other, rarer, cardiac diseases which may present in a similar fashion (e.g. atrial myxoma).

Initial assessment of mitral stenosis via the parasternal long axis window will reveal important information regarding the mitral valve, its associated apparatus and the left atrium. Mitral stenosis gives a characteristic "hockey stick" appearance to the anterior mitral valve leaflet (AMVL) as its body bows out during diastole but the tip is pulled in towards the posterior mitral valve leaflet (PMVL) by fusion at their commissures. This appearance is likened to a sail billowing in the wind (Figures 3.5.2, 3.5.3 and 3.5.4 normal, all on DVD).

M-mode imaging across the aortic valve allows measurement of the left atrial diameter, which is invariably large. This atrial dilatation renders patients highly susceptible to atrial fibrillation. This last feature can also be seen on M-mode imaging across the mitral valve leaflet tips.

There is a characteristic pattern to M-mode across the stenosed mitral valve. Normal mitral valve M-mode shows an M- and an W-shaped appearance to the AMVL and PMVL during diastole (Figure 3.5.5, on DVD). This represents the pattern of blood flow through the mitral valve, which is initially strong at the start of diastole, forcing both leaflets apart. The two leaflets gradually drift back together, but a second surge of blood, due to atrial systole, briefly pushes them apart again before valve closure occurs at the start of ventricular systole. In atrial fibrillation, this second surge of blood is lost. In mitral stenosis, instead of moving in opposite directions, the PMVL is pulled towards the AMVL as it opens at the start of diastole. As blood flow gradually lessens, the valves slowly return to the closed position, with or without the second push of atrial systole (Figure 3.5.6, on DVD).

The parasternal short axis window, at the mitral valve level, will further identify any calcification or fusion of the mitral valve cusps. There may be loss of the normal fish mouth appearance to the valvu-

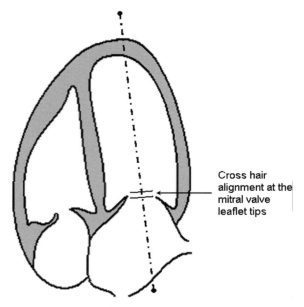

Figure 3.5.9 Apical 4 chamber showing the alignment of the cursor required for PWD imaging.

lar orifice (Figures 3.5.7 and 3.5.8 normal, all on DVD).

Changing to the apical 4/5 chamber window, it is again possible to see the mitral valvular movement pattern and any left atrial enlargement. Line up the cursor so that it transects the mitral valve and switch to pulsed wave Doppler imaging (Figure 3.5.9). Placing the cross-hairs of the cursor just at the tips of the valve leaflets will result in an image showing the pattern of blood flow through the mitral valve. This image will either be a single wave of variable dimensions if the patient is in atrial fibrillation, or a bifid consistent wave if sinus rhythm predominates (Figure 3.5.10, on DVD). The two peaks of the latter waveform represent firstly the initial filling of the left ventricle in diastole due to pulmonary pressure, and secondly filling due to atrial systole.

The flow of blood across the mitral valve can be used to estimate the area of the mitral valve orifice. Normal flow of blood across the valve has a rapid deceleration after peak velocity is reached, as

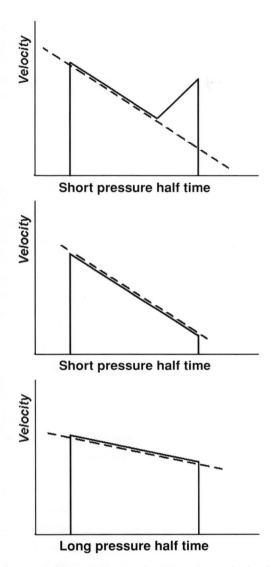

Figure 3.5.11 Appearance of PWD imaging at the level of the mitral valve leaflet tips in both mild and severe mitral stenosis.

Table 3.4. Mitral valve orifice area	
Severity of mitral stenosis	**Valve area (cm^2)**
Normal	4–6
Mild	2–4
Moderate	1–2
Severe	< 1

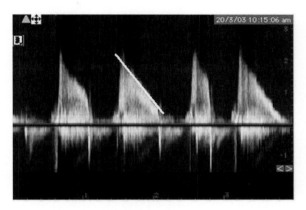

Figure 3.5.15 PWD imaging across the mitral valve in mild mitral stenosis with AF. Note that the stroke volume of each beat is different.

all blood is able to cross the valve quickly. However, with valvular obstruction the volume of blood which can cross the valve is limited, so a sustained high-velocity but low-volume jet occurs. These two appearances result in characteristic pulsed wave Doppler flow patterns, and can be further quantified by using the pressure half time tool (Figure 3.5.11). Mark the beginning of the (first) wave (A)

and its end point (B). From these variables the echo machine can calculate the mitral valve orifice area (Table 3.4).

This lady has mitral stenosis. She displays the characteristic appearance to her mitral valve leaflets in both the parasternal long axis and apical 4/5 chamber windows (Figures 3.5.12 and 3.5.13, both on DVD). The left atrium can also be seen to be enlarged. M-mode imaging across her mitral valve leaflet tips shows mitral stenosis with atrial fibrillation (Figure 3.5.14, on DVD). Her pulsed wave Doppler imaging of blood flow across the mitral valve shows the mitral stenosis to be mild (Figure 3.5.15). Her estimated mitral orifice cross-sectional area is 2 cm^2. This lady has mild to moderate mitral stenosis. She does not currently require intervention to her valve. Treatment of mitral stenosis can often be performed by balloon dilatation of the valve percutaneously, and open surgery is not always necessary.

Further examples

Figure 3.5.16 (on DVD) is of a left atrial myxoma. If this is large enough, it can also cause obstruction to mitral valve forwards flow (Figure 3.5.17, on DVD). Figure 3.5.18 (on DVD) shows another mass in the left atrium; a vegetation attached to the posterior leaflet of the mitral valve. This vegetation is due to bacterial endocarditis.

Case 6. Assessing the right heart

PowerPoint file: The use of ultrasound in diagnostic cardiology (CASE 6).

Scenario

A 65-year-old man is admitted for a left hemicolectomy to resect a sigmoid carcinoma. He is known to have chronic obstructive pulmonary disease, having smoked 20 cigarettes a day for 40 years. He is unable to walk further than 20 yards on the flat before breathlessness requires him to stop. Recently he has noticed that his ankles have become swollen, and his breathlessness is increasing.

On examination, his pulse is 80 beats per minute and is regular. Blood pressure is 110/85 mmHg. Saturations are 90% on air. He has a hyperexpanded, barrel-shaped chest. Heart sounds are normal. Chest auscultation reveals a global diffuse expiratory wheeze. He has pitting oedema to his ankles. ECG shows p-pulmonale and dominant r waves in V1 to V3. You wish to perform echocardiography.

Discussion

In this clinical situation it is uncertain whether this man has worsening SOB due to his pulmonary disease or undiagnosed heart failure. An echocardiogram will be able to assess both his right and left ventricular function. If right ventricular impairment is present, the source may be evident if related to the left ventricle (e.g. severe mitral regurgitation). However, echo is unable to differentiate primary lung disease (e.g. chronic obstructive pulmonary disease, COPD) from other condition which cause a raised pulmonary artery pressure (e.g. multiple pulmonary emboli). Alternative imaging techniques, such as CT pulmonary angiography, should be used in this case.

When assessing right ventricular function at echo, initially use the parasternal long axis window. This will show any dilatation to the right ventricular outflow tract, which is found at the apex of the image. Thickening of the right ventricular walls can also be seen, indicating hypertrophy. Rotating to the parasternal short axis view, at the level of the mitral valve apparatus, the right ventricle may be enlarged and of a similar shape and size to the left. Freeze this image and scroll through the cardiac cycle. In cases of right ventricular volume overload (i.e. severe tricuspid regurgitation), in diastole there may be a D-shape to the left ventricle. In severe right ventricular pressure overload (i.e. pulmonary hypertension), the left ventricle will have a D-shape in systole.

Stay with the parasternal short axis window and tilt the probe upwards to reveal the aortic valve, with the right heart surrounding it. Here the right atria and ventricle may be enlarged. Color flow Doppler imaging applied to this view may show a blue jet of tricuspid regurgitation. If located, this is often the best window in which to perform continuous wave Doppler measurement of the flow velocity of tricuspid regurgitation. The peak velocity of tricuspid regurgitation can then be converted to the pressure difference between the right atria and ventricle by using the simplified Bernoulli equation $\Delta P = 4V_{peak}^2$, see Case 3. If this pressure is added to the right atria pressure (which can be assessed by examining the jugular venous pressure) then an estimate of the pulmonary arterial pressure can be made.

(N.B. The pulmonary artery pressure is not a measure of the severity of tricuspid regurgitation, which is assessed by the same methods as used with mitral regurgitation.)

Next switch to the apical 4/5 chamber window or, if hyperinflated lungs obscure this view, the subcostal window. The features of right ventricular strain can be elicited again here and any tricuspid regurgitation present assessed.

This man has severe long-standing right heart strain, with a normal left heart. The parasternal long (Figures 3.6.1, 3.6.2 and 3.6.3 normal, all on DVD) and short axis (Figures 3.6.4, 3.6.5 and 3.6.6 normal, all on DVD) windows show a dilated right ventricle, with wall hypertrophy particularly evident in the long axis view. A continuous wave Doppler trace of his tricuspid regurgitation has a peak velocity of 3.5 m/s. The JVP was measured at 5 mmHg and therefore the estimated pulmonary artery pressure is approximately 50–60 mmHg (Figure 3.6.7, on DVD).

There is a characteristic D shape to the left ventricle during systole seen in the parasternal short axis window at the level of the mitral valve apparatus (Figures 3.6.8 and 3.6.9 normal, both on DVD). The apical 4 chamber window shows the right ventricle to be of similar size and structure to the left (Figures 3.6.10, 3.6.11 and 3.6.12 normal, all on DVD).

The most likely cause behind this echo appearance is chronic hypoxia secondary to COPD. However, other causes, such as a mediastinal lesion obstructing the pulmonary arteries, should be considered. The prognosis of these patients is poor, as pulmonary hypertension is a feature of end-stage COPD. The only treatment proven to be of benefit in these patients is long-term oxygen therapy. These factors all need to be taken into account when deciding upon this man's suitability for surgery.

Case 7. Assessing the pericardium

PowerPoint file: The use of ultrasound in diagnostic cardiology (CASE 7).

Scenario

A 45-year-old lady has breast cancer which has been in remission for 13 months. She has been admitted with an open fracture of her left humerus, sustained in a road traffic accident. She tells you that her breathing has been getting worse for a few weeks.

On examination she has a plethoric face. She is tachycardic with a pulse of 110 beats per minute. Her blood pressure is 95/60 mmHG. She is tachypnoeic at rest, with a respiratory rate of 24 per minute and oxygen saturations of 94% on air. She has quiet heart sounds with no murmurs. Her jugular venous pressure is raised at 8 cm above the sternal angle and appears fixed related to respiration. Chest auscultation is normal and no pedal edema is present. You wish to perform echocardiography.

Discussion

This is a clinical emergency. This lady has cardiac tamponade, most likely secondary to a paraneoplastic syndrome or malignant infiltration of the pericardium. The low blood pressure means that urgent drainage of the pericardial collection is required. Echocardiography will quickly confirm the diagnosis, and guide therapeutic aspiration.

Pericardial effusions can vary in size. Often acutely, the development of a few tens of milliliters is enough to cause tamponade. However, chronically very large effusions may develop with appropriate pericardial sack dilatation and therefore avoidance of tamponade. The major causes of pericardial effusions include trauma, TB, malignancy, heart failure, post-myocardial infarction, pericarditis, autoimmune, and post-cardiac surgery. A common cause in hospital is after the repositioning of a temporary pacing wire.

The key feature of a pericardial effusion to assess at echo is whether the right atrium collapses during diastole. This is because the right atrium acts as the weakest link of the cardiac circuit, being the point of lowest intrinsic pressure. As the pressure within the pericardial sack increases, this will therefore be the first point within the heart to become compressed.

This lady has a pericardial effusion, which is causing compression and near collapse of the right atrium during diastole (Figures 3.7.1, 3.7.2 and 3.7.3 normal, all on DVD). She requires urgent pericardiocentesis.

Case 8. Assessing simple congenital cardiac abnormalities

PowerPoint file: The use of ultrasound in diagnostic cardiology (CASE 8).

Scenario

A 26-year-old lady has been scheduled for routine abdominal laproscopic surgery to investigate chronic pelvic pain. She is otherwise fit and well.

On examination she has a regular pulse of 80 bpm and a blood pressure of 110/70 mmHg. She has a thrill palpable across her precordium, and a loud pan-systolic murmur radiating to her apex. Her JVP is not raised and her chest is clear to auscultation. You wish to perform echocardiography.

Discussion

The clinical vignette here is suggestive of a left to right intracardiac shunt, most likely a ventricular septal defect (VSD). This is arguably the commonest of all congenital heart malformations.

There are two main types of VSD: membranous and muscular (Figure 3.8.1, on DVD). The first type is a defect of the membranous portion of the interventricular septum, just behind the medial papillary muscle of the tricuspid valve. It may be associated with aortic regurgitation if the aortic valve structure is involved. The second type of VSD affects the muscular central part of the interventricular septum. This may also be a congenital anomaly or acquired during a septal infarction. Around 50% of VSDs close spontaneously, the smaller muscular variety being the most likely to do so.

Those defects which persist into adult life will be of variable significance according to their size and associated degree of left to right shunt. Echo is the ideal modality for both visualizing the site and size of the defect and also assessing the effect that it has had upon the left and right heart.

Starting in the parasternal long axis window, features of both left and right ventricular hypertrophy may be seen. A clear disruption to the septum may be evident with larger defects, as well as any associated ventricular wall aneurysm. Place color flow Doppler imaging across the septum and look for red flow towards the probe, indicating a left to right shunt in this view. An assessment of the size, position and degree of flow across the defect should be made, in a similar way to that used to assess regurgitate valves. To do this thoroughly involves examining the shunt in as many different planes as possible.

An estimate of the pulmonary artery pressure should also be performed. Methods outlined previously to do this are less accurate in the context of ventricular shunts, and a modified approach is needed. Firstly calculate the pressure difference between the left and right ventricle. This is done by measuring the peak VSD flow velocity, using continuous wave Doppler imaging as you would to assess aortic stenosis. Next use the modified Bernoulli equation to translate this value into a pressure difference. Now subtract this value from systolic brachial blood pressure measured with a sphygmomanometer, to give the right ventricular systolic pressure. This, in the absence of pulmonary stenosis, equates to pulmonary arterial pressure.

Pulmonary arterial pressure
$$= \text{systolic BP} - 4 \times \left(V_{\text{peak VSD}}\right)^2$$

The natural history of a significant VSD is towards an equilibration of left and right heart pressures with associated pulmonary hypertension and reversal of the intracardiac shunt (Eisenmenger's syndrome). Therefore knowledge of the pulmonary artery pressure is critical when deciding whether the defect requires closure, which can then be done either surgically or percutaneously.

The case outlined above is of a membranous VSD. At echo the defect is not immediately obvious in the parasternal long axis window, although significant left ventricular hypertrophy and right ventricular dilatation can be seen (Figures 3.8.2, 3.8.3 and 3.8.4 normal, all on DVD). The parasternal short axis also shows volume and pressure overload to the right ventricle, with a D-shaped left ventricle during the whole cardiac cycle (Figures 3.8.5, 3.8.6 and 3.8.7 normal, all on DVD). The apical 5 chamber view shows the defect well (Figures 3.8.8, 3.8.9 and 3.8.10 normal, all on DVD) and the left to right shunt of blood across it can be appreciated using color flow Doppler imaging (Figure 3.8.11, on DVD).

This lady requires a more detailed assessment of her VSD, to decide whether closure is required. She carries a risk of endocarditis and should receive antibiotic prophylaxis.

Further examples

Echo can also be used to assess for atrial septal defects (ASD), which are best visualized in the subcostal window. The commonest of these is a secundum type, which is in the center of the septum and may be associated with an atrial septal aneurysm (Figure 3.8.12, on DVD). A primum ASD is lower in the atrial septum, and may communicate with a high VSD (Figures 3.8.13 and 3.8.14, both on DVD). The assessment of other more complicated congenital cardiac malformations can also be performed at echo, but is outside the scope of this chapter.

FURTHER READING

Kaddoura S. *Echo Made Easy*. London, Churchill Livingstone, 2002.

Otto CM. *Textbook of Clinical Echocardiography*. 3rd edition. Philadelphia, Saunders, 2004.

Troianos CA. *Anesthesia for the Cardiac Patient*. Philadelphia, Mosby, 2004.

ACKNOWLEDGMENT

The author is grateful to Tony Bailey for the line illustrations.

Chapter 4

The role of echocardiography in the hemodynamically unstable patient in critical care and the operating theater

JULIAN SKOYLES AND HENRY SKINNER

Introduction

Echocardiography is becoming more accessible to anesthetists and intensivists. This interest has been driven principally through its role in cardiac surgery and adoption by cardiac anesthetists. There is strong evidence to support the use of transesophageal echocardiography (TEE) in the hemodynamically unstable patient, especially when the cause of instability is unclear [1]. The next decade should see a fall in the price of ultrasound machines and probes and so promote echocardiography as a valuable hemodynamic as well as diagnostic tool in all aspects of perioperative care.

The aim of this chapter is to outline the basic clinical roles for cardiac echocardiography in the unstable patient. Unless otherwise specified, the narrative and images refer to TEE, although many indications and views are in common with transthoracic echo (TTE). TTE is less invasive, but often can only provide limited information, as it relies on transthoracic windows that may be harder to obtain in ventilated or unstable patients. It is often undesirable to turn unstable or ventilated patients just to improve acoustic windows. Up to one half of critically ill ventilated patients in intensive care units cannot be adequately imaged by TTE, especially those requiring more than 10 cm positive end expiratory pressure (PEEP) [2]. Furthermore, many patients in intensive care units cannot be appropriately positioned, having sustained chest injury, or post-operative with dressings and tubes preventing adequate TTE. Because of these considerations, TEE has advantages (Table 4.1).

Recently, a simplified scheme has been published with a view to yielding maximum information from TTE in the critically ill but requiring minimal training (www.fate-protocol.com).

2D imaging in shock

Table 4.2 suggests some of the causes of shock encountered on an intensive care unit. The main advantage of echocardiography lies in the real-time 2D imaging of the heart and great vessels. In the majority of acute situations, it is sufficient to have this qualitative assessment in order to make an accurate diagnosis. The ability to identify structural causes of hypotension gives echocardiography an advantage over more conventional invasive hemodynamic monitoring, but it can also be used quantitatively to guide therapy. The majority of patients who are hemodynamically unstable have abnormalities of preload, cardiac contractility or afterload, all which can be assessed by echocardiography (Table 4.2).

Ultrasound in Anesthetic Practice, ed. Graham Arthurs and Barry Nicholls. Published by Cambridge University Press.
© Cambridge University Press 2009.

Table 4.1 Circumstances where the diagnostic yield of TEE is superior to TTE

Condition	Advantage of TEE
Mechanically ventilated patients	Absence of lung tissue between transducer and cardiac structures even in the presence of high airway pressures
Valvular vegetations	Better resolution of valve structures
Major pulmonary arterial emboli	Close proximity of esophagus to great vessels
Intracardiac emboli	Close proximity of esophagus to cardiac cavities, especially the left atrium
Aortic dissection	Superior views of the ascending and descending aorta, high sensitivity and specificity for diagnosis of aortic dissection*
Evaluation of native and prosthetic valves	Better resolution of native valves and the atrial side of prosthetic mitral valves

* Interposition of the right main bronchus between the esophagus and the distal part of the ascending aorta makes assessment of this area difficult.

Table 4.2 Conditions associated with hypotension where echocardiography can provide hemodynamic qualitative and, or quantitative data

Hypovolemia
Left ventricular failure
Right ventricular failure
Vasodilatation
Cardiac tamponade (2D and pulsed wave Doppler)
Acute valvular regurgitation (2D and color Doppler)
Aortic dissection

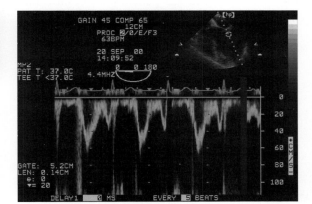

Figure 4.1 Normal diastolic flow through mitral valve.

Basic views

A comprehensive TEE study is recommended in every patient but falls beyond the scope of this text [3]. There are perhaps four fundamental views that could help in the initial assessment of the unstable patient.

The transgastric short axis view (TGSAX) of the left ventricle is central to the analysis of left ventricular filling and contractility (Figure 4.2, on DVD). It is unique in that it allows assessment of all three major coronary artery territories in a single view. This image is obtained by advancing the TEE probe 35–40 cm past the teeth into the stomach and flexing it slightly to ensure good contact with the diaphragm. Note that in the given example the left ventricle is

mildly hypertrophic (Figures 4.2 and 4.3, both on DVD).

The mid-esophageal four chamber view. This view is obtained by withdrawing the probe back into the esophagus 30–35 cm from the teeth with the scan plane 0°. This view shows all four cardiac chambers and in particular the septal and lateral walls of the left ventricle. It also demonstrates the anterior and posterior leaflets of the mitral valve on the left and right of the image, respectively. Flow through the mitral valve is parallel to the ultrasound beam, and makes this image suitable for Doppler assessment of mitral inflow or color Doppler to assess mitral regurgitation. Figure 4.1 shows normal diastolic flow through the mitral valve with the sample volume positioned at the leaflet tips. Flow towards the transducer is depicted above the baseline and flow away from the transducer appears below.

The mid-esophageal two chamber view (Figure 4.4, on DVD). In this image, the position of the probe is unchanged but the scan plane rotated forwards to 90° to show the left atrium and left ventricle. The left atrial appendage and anterior ventricular wall appears on the right of the screen and the inferior ventricular wall on the left of the screen. An accurate assessment of ventricular volume can be made from this image, as it shows both the length and width of the left ventricle. In this patient there is moderate impairment of the left ventricle.

The mid-esophageal long axis view (Figure 4.5, on DVD). The scan plane is further rotated to 120° to reveal the anteroseptal ventricular wall and part of the right ventricular outflow tract on the right. The posterior left ventricular wall is on the left of the screen. It also demonstrates the mitral valve (the anterior leaflet is now displayed on the right side in close association with the aortic root), the left ventricular outflow tract, and the aortic valve in its long axis.

Assessment of preload

Echocardiography is superior to pulmonary capillary wedge pressures in representing preload, especially at the extremes of preload. Preload can be estimated by tracing the endocardial border in the TGSAX view during diastole; the end-diastolic area (EDA). The normal range is 10–20 cm^2.

Software on most machines allows calculation of left ventricular volume (35–75 ml/m^2) by tracing the inner border of the left ventricular cavity in the mid-esophageal two chamber view.

Preload can also be gauged by measuring blood flow velocities across the mitral valve that is related to an atrial ventricular pressure gradient in diastole. Pulsed wave Doppler through the mitral valve can give characteristic flow patterns related to preload and ventricular diastolic performance.

Low preload is found in hypovolemia due to any cause such as bleeding, burns or sepsis. Figure 4.6 (on DVD) demonstrates a TGSAX view in a hypovolemic patient. There is almost obliteration of the ventricular cavity during systole with "kissing" of the papillary muscles. Figure 4.7 (on DVD) demonstrates the effect of fluid resuscitation in the same patient, and confirms the value of repeat assessments to guide further therapy. When a patient remains hypotensive after a fluid challenge, a real-time image of the state of ventricular filling is informative.

High preload may be seen in the failing ventricle (Figure 4.8, on DVD), especially with over-zealous fluid resuscitation. This patient should benefit from vasodilators, diuretics and possible inotropic support.

TTE or TEE may help to define problems in patients even when there is constant monitoring of pulmonary artery pressures. Echocardiography has been shown to be more reliable than Swan–Ganz catheter pressure in determining the cause of hypotension [4].

Other causes of a low output state

Cardiac tamponade (Figure 4.9, on DVD) occurs when the intrapericardial pressure, normally sub-atmospheric, exceeds the intracardiac pressure. On 2D there is typically early diastolic collapse of the right ventricle and late diastolic collapse of the right atrium that is restored after drainage of the effusion (Figure 4.10, on DVD). Under physiological conditions there is equal variation in intrapericardial and intrathoracic pressures during the respiratory cycle. With tamponade there is a lesser fall in intrapericardial pressure during inspiration (during expiration in a ventilated patient) causing a reduction between the diastolic pressure gradient between pulmonary capillaries and the left ventricle. This manifests in a greater than 25% variation of early mitral inflow velocities (E wave) between inspiration and expiration.

Valve dysfunction

Chronic significant aortic and mitral regurgitation lead to volume overload and impairment of left ventricular function. There is often associated left atrial dilatation. Acute mitral regurgitation may follow a ruptured papillary muscle or chordae tendinea. The 4 chamber mid-esophageal view (Figure 4.11, on DVD) shows prolapse of the posterior mitral leaflet. The leaflets fail to coapt, resulting in severe mitral regurgitation represented by the green turbulent jet on color flow Doppler (Figure 4.12, on DVD). There is less time for atrial compensatory enlargement resulting in pulmonary venous congestion.

Acute mitral regurgitation is also a complication of infective endocarditis, and patients may become unstable due to acute left ventricular failure with or without pulmonary edema and perhaps accompanying sepsis.

Acute aortic regurgitation can be caused by infective endocarditis or ascending aortic dissection. Figure 4.13 (on DVD) demonstrates a large vegetation on the non-coronary aortic cusp, and Figure 4.14 (on DVD) shows clearly a dissection flap in the ascending aorta. This patient has severe aortic regurgitation because of prolapse of an aortic cusp and disruption of the aortic root anatomy by the dissection. Because the thoracic aorta is so close to the esophagus, TEE has 99% sensitivity and 90% specificity for suspected aortic dissection [5]. In addition, the procedure avoids the transfer of unstable patients into CT scans. These patients may decompensate from acute increase in preload and can have features of hypovolemia, hemopericardium or myocardial ischemia if the coronary ostia are involved in the dissection. TEE should establish the entry site of the dissection, assess the aortic valve for involvement and establish the presence of effusions and tamponade.

More subtle degrees of valvular regurgitation are not uncommon in the critically ill and experienced judgment is required. However, hemodynamically significant gross regurgitant valve lesions can be readily appreciated with minimal training. Mild tricuspid regurgitation is a common finding in the normal population, but more significant tricuspid regurgitation can be secondary to increased pulmonary arterial pressures and right ventricular dilatation in a critically ill patient. The TGSAX (Figure 4.15, on DVD) shows an example of a patient with acute right ventricular failure due to a pulmonary embolus. Note the profound increase in right ventricular size compared to the left ventricle. In the critically ill patient without myocardial infarction, valve dysfunction, left ventricular impairment or known pulmonary disease, the finding of right ventricular dilatation or hypokinesis indicates a high probability of pulmonary embolism. Patients with a large main pulmonary thrombus may occasionally be diagnosed by TEE alone, but spiral CT has a greater sensitivity [6].

Assessment of left ventricular contractility

The TGSAX view (Figure 4.2, on DVD) demonstrates, clockwise from the top, the mid segments of the inferior, posterior, lateral, anterior, antero-septal and septal walls, respectively. It does not show the basal (towards the mitral valve) and apical segments of these walls. There are six basal segments described and four apical segments (the antero-septal and posterior walls do not have apical segments). The other three views must also be scrutinized to assess all 16 segments.

Normal myocardium will both radially shorten and thicken in systole. Any reduction of this thickening is highly sensitive for ischemia and precedes ECG changes. With complete absence of coronary flow the myocardium thins during systole. Each segment can be described as normal, hypokinetic, severely hypokinetic or akinetic. A dyskinetic segment thins and bulges outwards during systole. Figure 4.16 (on DVD) demonstrates a patient with inferior wall hypokinesis towards the top of the image suggestive of an acute ischemic event.

Experienced ultrasonographers can simply eye-ball the four views and then estimate an ejection fraction to assess global systolic function. The TGSAX view can also be used to quantify ventricular performance. The fractional area change represents the contractility in two dimensions. It is calculated by measuring areas traced around the endocardial borders on a recorded cycle in both systole and diastole (Diagram 4.1, Table 4.3).

Measurement of cardiac output with echocardiography

The use of Doppler modes in echocardiography allows velocities to be measured. The stroke volume can be calculated by tracing the mitral inflow velocity at the level of the mitral valve annulus during diastole. The software integrates this to produce a "stroke distance", i.e. the distance red cells have traveled through the mitral annulus. Assuming a circular geometry of the mitral annulus, the cross-sectional area is calculated by measuring the diameter. The product of this area and the stroke distance is the stroke volume. Cardiac output is calculated by multiplying in the stroke volume by the heart rate.

Stroke volume can also be calculated by subtracting the end systolic volume from the end diastolic volume. These methods are rarely used in the acute setting, as they are time-consuming. However, they are valuable for later "off-line" calculations.

Assessment of afterload

Patients may become hypotensive due to reductions in afterload caused by volatile or intravenous anesthetic agents, vasodilators or low systemic vascular resistance in septic shock. However, there are some important causes of hypotension that are associated with an increased afterload. The most

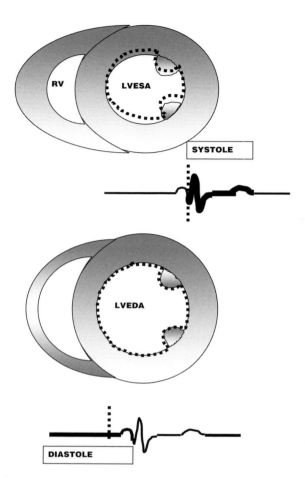

Deep Transgastric Short Axis Ventricular (TGSAX) view with Transesophageal Echo

Fractional Area Change can be used to estimate Left Ventricular Ejection Fraction (LVEF)

$$\text{Fractional area change} = \frac{\text{LVEDA} - \text{LVESA}}{\text{LVEDA}}$$

Normal range 40–70%
One should realize that the TGSAX view shows only the mid segments and errors could be made if significant wall motion abnormalities exist in basal or apical segments.

Diagram 4.1   LVEDA = left ventricular end diastolic area; LVESA = left ventricular end systolic area.

common is severe aortic stenosis with reduced leaflet separation and turbulence beyond the aortic valve in the mid-esophageal long axis view (Figure 4.17, on DVD). This view is important to assess left

Table 4.3 Quantifiable changes in left ventricle end-diastolic area (LVEDA) and left ventricle end systolic area (LVESA) in hypotensive state

Condition	EDA*	ESA**	FAC***
Hypovolemia	Decreased	Decreased	Increased
Poor ventricular function	Increased	Increased	Decreased
Vasodilatation	Normal	Decreased	Increased

*EDA, end diastolic area; **ESA, end systolic area; ***FAC, fractional area change.

ventricular outflow tract obstruction as seen in hypertrophic obstructive cardiomyopathy. Rarely, the cause of outflow tract obstruction is systolic anterior motion of the anterior leaflet of the mitral valve (Figure 4.18, on DVD), as seen in this patient with hypertrophic obstructive cardiomyopathy. Note that during systole the anterior mitral leaflet (on the right) is sucked into the outflow tract causing a dynamic obstruction with turbulence in the outflow tract and concomitant mitral regurgitation. Abnormal systolic anterior motion of the mitral valve has been described with other causes of left ventricular hypertrophy and is also a recognized complication of mitral valve repair. Here the immediate treatment is fluid resuscitation, vasoconstrictors and even beta blockers to keep the outflow tract open before mitral valve surgery is contemplated.

In summary, 2D, Doppler and color echocardiography are valuable in delineating pathology and hemodynamics in the critically ill or injured patient and in certain perioperative situations. TEE appears to have distinct advantages in certain settings.

REFERENCES

1. Cheitlin MD, Armstrong WF, Aurigemma GP, *et al.* ACC/AHA/ASE 2003 Guideline update for the clinical application of echocardiography: Summary article. *Journal of the American Society of Echocardiography* 2003;16:1091–110.

2. Parker MM, Cunnion RE, Parrillo JE. Echocardiography and nuclear cardiac imaging in the critical care unit. *Journal of American Medical Association* 1985;254:2935–9.

3. Shanewise J, Cheung AT, Aronson S, *et al.* ASE/SCA guidelines for performing a comprehensive intraoperative multiplane transesophageal echocardiography examination. *Anesthesia and Analgesia* 1999;89:870–84.

4. Heidenreich PA, Stainback RF, Redberg RF, *et al.* Transesophageal echocardiography predicts mortality in critically ill patients with unexplained hypotension. *Journal of American College of Cardiology* 1995;26:152–8.

5. Keren A, Kim CB, Hu BS. Accuracy of multiplane and biplane transoesophageal echocardiography in diagnosis of typical acute aortic dissection and intramural haematoma. *Journal of the American College of Cardiologists* 1996;28:627–36.

6. Pruszczyk P, Torbicki A, Pacho R, *et al.* Noninvasive diagnosis of suspected severe pulmonary embolism: transesophageal echocardiography vs spiral CT. *Chest* 1997;112:722–8.

Chapter 5

Transesophageal diagnostic Doppler monitoring

ROBERT KONG

Introduction

Over the last decade, the use of the pulmonary artery flotation catheter for cardiac output monitoring has declined. In contrast, less-invasive techniques such as the esophageal Doppler are becoming the predominant methods for hemodynamic monitoring in the intensive care unit. Several studies now show that the outcome of patients undergoing major surgery can be improved with "goal-directed" intraoperative fluid management [1]. Most of these studies have used the esophageal Doppler and undoubtedly this is a factor accounting for the increased interest in esophageal Doppler monitoring during surgery.

Blood flow velocity is measured in the descending thoracic aorta by an ultrasound (Doppler) transducer mounted on the end of a probe. The esophageal Doppler provides an estimate of cardiac output and, in addition, analysis of the aortic velocity waveform gives an indication of cardiac contractility as well as intravascular volume status.

Some clinicians may be familiar with the Hemosonic (Arrow International, USA) or TECO (Medicina, UK) esophageal Doppler devices. However, the CardioQ (Deltex Medical, Chichester, UK) has the biggest user base in the UK and continental Europe. The same company also brought out the ODM II, which was replaced by the CardioQ in 1999.

This chapter and the accompanying video aim to give a comprehensive overview of the CardioQ and provide a practical guide for novice users.

The CardioQ

The components of the CardioQ are the monitor, the esophageal probe and the patient interface cable that connects the probe to the monitor.

The monitor

Measuring $32 \times 15 \times 26$ cm, the monitor weighs about 5.4 kg. The outer casing is made of a hard polycarbonate. A handle is built into the upper edge of the box and a custom-made hook can be used to suspend the monitor from here to (for example) an IV pole. There are two rotary dials on the front of the machine. The smaller, upper one is used to adjust the volume of the sound coming through a single speaker. The lower, larger dial has different functions, such as altering the electronic gain of the signal or selecting variables for display depending on the page displayed on the 10 inch LCD screen. Six buttons are located on the lower front edge of the box below the screen and correspond to the menu options shown on the screen (Figure 5.1).

Ultrasound in Anesthetic Practice, ed. Graham Arthurs and Barry Nicholls. Published by Cambridge University Press.
© Cambridge University Press 2009.

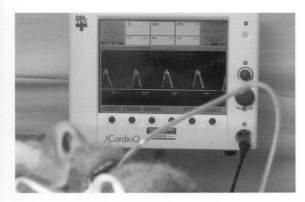

Figure 5.1 CardioQ monitor displaying aortic waveform in Probe Focus mode.

Doppler probe

The esophageal probe consists of a piezo-electric crystal (the ultrasound transducer) mounted at one end of a 0.5 m length of steel spring. The entire length is encased in a clear silicone covering which extends beyond the spring at the other end to incorporate a connector for the patient interface cable. At the transducer end, the tip is moulded to a 45° bevel, which defines the assumed angle of insonation relative to the axis of the descending aorta. The probe has an outer diameter of approximately 19 Fr (6.3 mm).

The design of the probe allows it to be rigid but flexible and enables the distal tip (transducer) to be rotated by holding and twisting the probe at its proximal end.

There are three depth markers on the current adult probes, positioned at 35, 40 and 45 cm from the distal end (Figure 5.2, on DVD). Versions of the adult probes differ in the pre-programmed maximum monitoring duration from 6, 12 or 240 h. Another version of the adult probe can be distinguished by the opaque, white silicone encasing the entire length of the probe. This probe is programmed for a 10-day monitoring limit and has two movable markers set at 35 and 40 cm. The Awake Doppler probe has a more flexible spring and is designed specifically for nasal insertion, although all the probes can be inserted orally or through the nose. The Pediatric probe (KDP 72) has a similar construction, but is shorter and has markings from 15 to 40 cm at 5 cm intervals. This probe has a monitoring limit of 72 h and can be used in children weighing upwards of 3 kg. All the probes are for single patient use only.

Patient data

Once the probe is connected to the monitor, via the patient interface cable, the screen shows the Patient Data page. The patient's age, weight and height are entered here for the nomogram (see later). Subsequently, pressing the *Accept Data* key will store this information in the probe (in the chip at the connector). If the probe has already been used in a patient, the stored data will be displayed. In clinical practice, the patient's weight and height may not be readily available. If this is the case, it is worth noting that age is the most important variable, although a reasonable estimate of weight and height will improve the accuracy of cardiac output determination. For the pediatric nomogram, a reliable patient height (length) is essential.

Probe insertion

The lubricated probe can be inserted into the esophagus via the mouth or nose. It is necessary only to apply a generous blob of aqueous lubricant to the tip of the probe. The gel also acts as a coupling agent to improve signal detection. The direction of the bevel is not important, but of course care must be taken not to traumatize the turbinates if nasal insertion is attempted. It is often simpler to insert the probe into the approximate depth, and at a convenient moment later connect it to the monitor.

The descending aorta is located postero-lateral to the esophagus (Figure 5.3). With the monitor set to *Probe Focus* mode, the aortic flow signal should be searched by rotating the probe to the patient's left or right and by advancing or retracting the probe about 1 cm at a time (Figure 5.4, on DVD).

Table 5.1 Guide for pediatric esophageal Doppler probe insertion

Patient length (cm)	Doppler depth (cm)	Probe marker position (cm)
50–55	15–17	Between 15 and 20
56–60	17–20	Between 15 and 20
61–70	16–23	Between 15 and 25
71–80	17–24	Between 15 and 25
81–100	19–28	Between 15 and 30
101–120	24–28	Between 20 and 30
121–140	27–34	Between 25 and 35
>140	27–40	Between 25 and 40

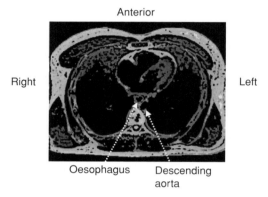

Figure 5.3 Sketch showing relationship of esophagus to descending aorta.

In adults of average height, the aortic signal is usually found when the probe, inserted orally, is at a depth of 35–40 cm at the lips. For the nasal route, the probe should be advanced a further 5 cm. As a general guide, the depth of insertion is correlated with the height of the patient: push the probe in more or less if the patient is taller or shorter than average. It would be unusual, however, to find the aortic signal at insertion depths of less than 30 cm or more than 45 cm at the lips. For pediatric patients, the depth of insertion should be guided by the patient's length (Table 5.1).

Signal acquisition

Correct identification of the descending aortic waveform is a prerequisite for esophageal Doppler

monitoring. After processing by Fast Fourier Transform, blood flow waveform is represented on the monitor as a spectral display of the distribution of red blood cell flow velocities (vertical axis) against time (horizontal axis). In contrast to standard echocardiography Doppler convention, the CardioQ displays velocities moving away from the transducer as a positive signal (above the line), and as a negative signal (below the line) if blood flow is towards the transducer. In other words, descending aortic blood flow is shown as a signal above the line.

The descending aortic waveform

The most frequent fault observed in novice users is related to obtaining the descending aortic flow waveform. This waveform is approximately triangular in shape, above the line and pulsatile, occurring predominantly during systole. There may be a very low velocity positive (forward) flow during all or part of diastole (Figure 5.5).

Some negative flow in early diastole is occasionally seen. In the *Probe Focus* mode, the user should try to obtain a waveform where the brightest signal (orange to white color when the gain is appropriately adjusted) is on the periphery of the triangle. In the optimal waveform, the center of the triangle is relatively dark. These characteristics

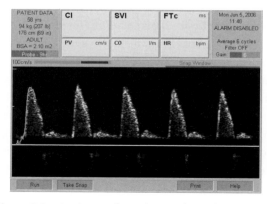

Figure 5.5 Aortic waveform showing low velocity forward flow in diastole.

can be observed in the waveform on the monitor (Figure 5.1). Three features should be borne in mind in trying to obtain an optimal waveform:

(1) See – a characteristic waveform image on screen (as described above).
(2) Sound – clear and whip-like pulsatile sound.
(3) Velocity – waveform with the highest peak velocity.

A useful tip is to try, initially, to concentrate on the sound only by adjusting the probe without looking at the screen. Many novice users find that in this way, identifying the "best" signal is really quite easy. The monitor has a facility to help identify the highest peak velocity by pressing the *Show PVD* button. This initiates a blue line that automatically identifies and stays at the level of the highest velocity. Some clinicians, however, simply eyeball the varying heights of the waveforms. Turbulent flow or poor alignment of the probe (relative to the descending aorta) is likely to lead to spectral dispersion (Figure 5.6, on DVD), which should warn against accepting the absolute flow and flow-derived values given by the monitor.

Other waveforms

The only cardiac valvular abnormality that impinges on the descending aortic waveform is moderate to severe aortic regurgitation when there is the presence of diastolic flow reversal (Figure 5.7, on DVD). Severe aortic stenosis with impaired contractility may result in a damped, dome-shaped (rather than triangular) waveform (Figure 5.8, on DVD).

Only the celiac axis waveform is likely to be mistaken for descending aorta and produce completely erroneous data (Figure 5.9, on DVD). Characteristically, the upright waveform of the celiac axis has a significant diastolic velocity that should not be present in the descending aorta. Signals from other vessels are usually very different and unlikely to be confused with the descending aortic waveform (e.g. intracardiac signal as in Figure 5.10, on DVD). Pulmonary artery waveform is displayed below the line

and also has two distinct components – systolic and diastolic flow (Figure 5.11, on DVD).

The nomogram

As the CardioQ measures blood flow velocity, cardiac output has to be derived. Theoretically, left ventricular stroke volume could be obtained from the "stroke distance" if the cross-sectional area of the aorta at the point of measurement, as well as the proportion of left ventricular stroke volume that arrives at the descending aorta, are known. The stroke distance is obtained by measuring the velocity–time integral (area under the curve) of each aortic waveform. Calculating the cardiac output in this way, however, has the potential for significant errors. But the theoretical validity of this approach has given rise to a common misconception that the nomogram (obtained from the age, weight and height) gives the patient's aortic diameter or cross-sectional area. In fact, the nomogram was empirically derived in a cohort of patients simultaneously monitored with an esophageal Doppler device and a pulmonary artery catheter, from which cardiac output was measured by thermodilution. Thus a true measured aortic velocity (giving stroke distance), from a suitable aortic waveform, can be related to stroke volume. That this nomogram is an acceptable calibration factor for obtaining stroke volume from the esophageal Doppler is confirmed by several comparison (validation) studies between esophageal Doppler and pulmonary artery catheter, as well as by more than a decade of clinical experience [2]. The limits of the nomogram for

Table 5.2 Nomogram for age, weight and height limits of adult and pediatric patients		
	Adult	**Pediatric**
Age (years)	16–99	0–15
Weight (kg)	30–150	3–60
Height (cm)	149–212	50–170

Table 5.3 Normal hemodynamic ranges

Stroke volume Index (SVI) (ml/m²)	Cardiac Index (CI) (l/min/m²)	Peak velocity (PV) Age(years)	(cm/s)
35–65	3.5–4.5*	∼ 20	90–120
		∼ 50	70–100
		∼ 70	50–80

Note: "Low cardiac output syndrome" can be defined as CI ≤ 2.5 l/(min m²).

adults and pediatric patients (which were derived separately) are shown in Table 5.2.

Measuring the waveform

When the correct and best waveform has been located, the gain should be altered using the larger dial. The *Auto Gain* facility will adjust the gain automatically, but it is probably simpler to adjust the dial manually: the gain should be neither too high nor too low! At this point, pressing the *Run* button will initiate a green line to envelope the waveform. Within a few beats, if the signal is stable, small white triangles will mark the start and end of each waveform and an arrow will show the peak velocity. The parameters chosen for display will then appear on the upper part of the screen (Figure 5.12, on DVD). The values will refresh at a rate ranging from beat-to-beat to every 20 cardiac cycles. An averaging rate of 5 cycles is sufficient for sinus rhythm, but a rate of at least 10 cycles should be used when monitoring patients in atrial fibrillation.

One final and critical check should be made at this stage. Ensure that the green line faithfully outlines the limits and the triangles accurately pinpoint the start and end of the waveform (Figure 5.13, on DVD). A poor quality signal and excessive or inadequate gain adjustment can lead to a mismatch between the waveform and the green line. As the various parameters are computed by the position of the green line and the markers, any measurement will be inaccurate if these conditions are not met.

Cardiac output

Cardiac output is obtained from the product of stroke volume and heart rate. As the normal resting cardiac output is related to the size of the patient (approximately 0.1 l/(min kg)), cardiac index and stroke volume index – obtained from cardiac output or stroke volume divided by body surface area – are arguably more useful in the clinic. Body surface area is calculated from height and weight (Dubois formula). Table 5.3 shows some normal ranges for cardiac and stroke volume index in adults.

Flow time-corrected (FTc)

Descending aortic flow occurs during systole, which occupies approximately one-third of the cardiac cycle. One would expect, therefore, a flow time of approximately 333 ms at a heart rate of 60 beats per minute. The absolute flow time is heart rate-dependent and will increase or decrease if the heart rate is slower or faster than 60/min, respectively. But flow time is also influenced by loading conditions on the heart – preload and afterload – and, to some extent, contractility. A more useful hemodynamic indicator is obtained if the effect of heart rate on flow time could be "eliminated". As heart rate increases, the duration of diastole as a proportion of each cardiac cycle will decrease. Thus correction of systolic flow time interval for heart rate – analogously to the correction of ECG intervals for heart rate – leads to the Flow Time-corrected (FTc) parameter. The normal range for this is 330–360 ms. Consequently, irrespective of heart rate, the FTc can be used as a quick guide to the underlying hemodynamic condition.

Abnormal FTc situations

FTc < 330 ms

(1) In the majority of cases in perioperative monitoring, a low FTc is indicative of low intravascular volume. The accompanying stroke volume index is typically low also (but not necessarily): a fluid challenge results in an immediate increase in stroke volume and FTc (Figure 5.14). It is common practice to consider a stroke volume increase of at least 10% as indicating preload-responsiveness. Failure to increase the stroke volume by 10% after the fluid challenge suggests that either the preload limit has been reached or an alternative etiology should be considered if the FTc remains low (Figure 5.15, on DVD).

(2) The FTc may be low because of impaired left ventricular function (systolic or diastolic or both). In such cases, the peak velocity (see below) will also be decreased. Impaired right ventricular function or any obstruction to right to left flow, e.g. pulmonary embolus, can result in a low FTc because of reduced left ventricular preload (Figure 5.16, on DVD).

(3) Some clinicians consider that a low FTc is a result of an increased afterload. Other than in iatrogenic cases (e.g. inappropriate admin-

istration of norepinephrine), however, this is probably in reference to the peripheral vasoconstriction that may be seen in response to hypovolemia or cardiac failure.

FTc > 360 ms

(1) Prolonged FTc indicates a condition of low afterload – peripheral vasodilatation, which may be due to any one or more clinical factors (e.g. sepsis, vasodilating drugs, anesthesia or epidural). Typically, the associated stroke volume in the adequately resuscitated patient will be high (Figure 5.17, on DVD). Occasionally, as in severe sepsis, there may be concurrent myocardial dysfunction and the cardiac output may be in the normal range.

Peak velocity

Peak velocity (cm/s) is influenced by both loading conditions and left ventricular contractility. Myocardial contractility decreases with aging and this is the principal explanation for the reduction in the measured peak velocity in older patients (Table 5.3). Changes in left ventricular contractility as a result of pathology or drug therapy would be reflected by changes in peak velocities. In general, an increase in preload as well as a decrease in afterload will lead to a rise in peak velocity. Conversely, peak velocity decreases when preload is low or afterload is high. When the aortic waveform signal is sub-optimal, the measured peak velocity will be lower than expected and stroke volume will be underestimated.

Mean acceleration

The mean acceleration (m/s^2) is the average rate of change of velocity of blood flow from the beginning of the waveform until the time on reaching peak velocity. Mean acceleration reflects left ventricular contractility and to a lesser extent afterload and preload. The load-dependence of mean acceleration should caution against the use of this

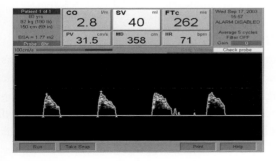

Figure 5.14 Effect of fluid resuscitation in a hypovolemic patient.

parameter as a direct indicator of left ventricular contractility in individual patients. Across patients, however, low mean acceleration tends to suggest reduced contractility.

Which parameters?

Esophageal Doppler monitoring provides a rich source of hemodynamic information. The shape of the aortic waveform alone gives a clue to the underlying hemodynamic condition even before the quantitative data are considered. Clinicians may be overwhelmed by the numerous (11!) parameters offered by the CardioQ; 6 are displayed at any one time. The surfeit of data leads to confusion about how they should be integrated for decision-making. The author's advice is to restrict data interpretation, initially, to flow time-corrected, stroke volume index and cardiac index. These three parameters immediately provide information on global blood flow and the likeliest underlying hemodynamic abnormality. This gives the clinician a starting point from which to assess the effect of further therapy. Ignoring peak velocity and mean acceleration during the learning phase of the CardioQ will not significantly limit its utility. Of course, incorporating them into the analysis may prove to be essential in more complex situations.

Indications for CardioQ monitoring

Several prospective randomized controlled trials support the use of esophageal Doppler monitoring to guide fluid management during major surgery or in the immediate postoperative period [3–7]. The strategy has been referred to as "goal-directed", in that the objective has been to titrate fluid boluses to obtain the highest achievable stroke volume during surgery. Some studies have also added inotropic agents, but these do not appear to be essential [8]. It is not clear what mechanism is at play, but the studies all show reductions in post-operative complications and length of hospital stay when compared to standard care. Therefore, a clear indication

for esophageal Doppler monitoring would be in major general, colorectal, hip and cardiac surgery [9]. At present, there are no studies that have evaluated esophageal Doppler monitoring in day-case or surgery of short duration when minimal blood or fluid loss would be expected.

Cardiac output is frequently measured in intensive care patients. However, there is little evidence to show that this has any impact on patient outcome, irrespective of the type of cardiac output monitor – including the esophageal Doppler [10]. Nevertheless, if the intention is simply to monitor physiological changes, the esophageal Doppler provides a tool to do that with virtually no associated risk. In trauma patients, esophageal Doppler-guided resuscitation has been shown to result in better outcomes [11].

The following considerations may influence clinicians to choose esophageal Doppler monitoring over other technologies:

(1) It avoids the need for central venous or arterial access.
(2) Hemodynamic data are usually obtained rapidly.
(3) Nursing staff can use the technology to facilitate early diagnosis and treatment.
(4) It is easy to transport the monitor to other clinical areas within a hospital.
(5) There is no suitable alternative monitoring in some types of surgery.
(6) Awake patients can be monitored relatively quickly and easily.

Limitations

After appropriate training and experience, clinicians should expect to fail only rarely to obtain the aortic signal. To ensure that the optimal waveform is being recorded, the probe position should be checked before each measurement. Clinicians regard this as a major limitation of this device, preferring the simplicity of other technologies that continuously display the cardiac output value. But with practice, a brief probe "check" can be integrated into the procedure for esophageal Doppler use. It is often assumed that the presence of other devices in the esophagus (e.g. nasogastric tube) will interfere with signal acquisition. This has not been the author's experience, although this should be considered if a satisfactory signal is elusive. Esophageal Doppler monitoring is not recommended in patients with significant pathology of the esophagus or who are undergoing pharyngo-esophageal surgery. Monitoring is unreliable or impossible in some conditions – aortic dissection (turbulent flow and interference due to the intimal flap), during cross clamping of descending aorta, and concurrent intra-aortic balloon pump.

Conclusion

Esophageal Doppler monitoring provides a safe technique for assessing a range of hemodynamic conditions as well as a tool to guide fluid therapy. The skills needed to use this device (CardioQ) can be acquired in a short time. Aside from some limitations, esophageal Doppler monitoring has not been associated with any important adverse effects. A growing evidence base supports esophageal Doppler use to guide intraoperative fluid management with the potential to improve patient outcome in major surgery.

REFERENCES

1. Tote SP, Grounds RM. Performing perioperative optimization of the high-risk surgical patient. *British Journal of Anaesthesia* 2006;97:4–11.
2. Cholley BP, Singer M. Esophageal Doppler: non-invasive cardiac output monitor. *Echocardiography* 2003;20:763–9.
3. Sinclair S, James S, Singer M. Intraoperative intravascular volume optimisation and length of hospital stay after repair of proximal femoral fracture: randomised controlled trial. *British Medical Journal* 1997;315:909–12.
4. Gan TJ, Soppitt A, Maroof M, et al. Goal-directed intraoperative fluid administration reduces length of hospital stay after major surgery. *Anesthesiology* 2002;97: 820–6.
5. Venn R, Steele A, Richardson P, Poloniecki J, Grounds M, Newman P. Randomized controlled trial to investigate influence of the fluid challenge on duration of hospital stay and perioperative morbidity in patients with hip fractures. *British Journal of Anaesthesia* 2002;88:65–71.
6. Wakeling HG, McFall MR, Jenkins CS, et al. Intraoperative oesophageal Doppler guided fluid management shortens postoperative hospital stay after major bowel surgery. *British Journal of Anaesthesia* 2005;95:634–42.
7. Noblett SE, Snowden CP, Shenton BK, Horgan AF. Randomised clinical trial assessing the effect of Doppler-optimized fluid management on outcome after elective colorectal resection. *British Journal of Surgery* 2006;93:1069–76.
8. Stone MD, Wilson RJT, Cross J, Williams BT. Effect of adding dopexamine to intraoperative volume expansion in patients undergoing major elective abdominal surgery. *British Journal of Anaesthesia* 2003;91:619–24.
9. McKendry M, McGloin H, Saberi D, Caudwell L, Brady AR, Singer M. Randomised controlled trial assessing the impact of a nurse delivered, flow monitored protocol for optimisation of circulatory status after cardiac surgery. *British Medical Journal* 2004;329:258–62.
10. Harvey S, Harrison DA, Singer M, *et al.* Assessment of the clinical effectiveness of pulmonary artery catheters in management of

patients in intensive care (PAC-Man): a randomised controlled trial. *Lancet* 2005;366:472–7.

11. Chytra I, Pradl R, Bosman R, Pelnar P, Kasal E, Zidkova A. Esophageal Doppler-guided fluid management decreases blood lactate levels in multiple-trauma patients: a randomized controlled trial. *Critical Care* 2007;11:R24.

Chapter 6

Use of ultrasound in the intensive care unit

JOHN ORAM AND ANDREW BODENHAM

Introduction

Over the last decade, ultrasound scanners have become cheaper and smaller and have increasingly been used by clinicians with no formal radiology training. In the intensive care unit (ICU) these devices have become commonplace for line insertion, but as clinical experience grows the range of applications for ultrasound in the modern ICU has expanded [1–5]. In the hands of intensivists, ultrasound has been used to guide needle drainage procedures and percutaneous tracheostomy, and to aid in the diagnosis of pleural, pulmonary and abdominal conditions.

The range of procedures which can be attempted by individual intensivists varies greatly. Some will use ultrasound only for line insertions, whilst others are regularly performing diagnostic scanning and deep drainage procedures. This increased use is now being recognized and formal training and accreditation has been recommended [6].

This chapter is concerned with simple techniques which will be useful and accessible to all; we will not concentrate on ultrasound-based monitoring devices (such as transcranial and esophageal Doppler).

Equipment

A range of ultrasound machines are available: some of these are small units designed purely for vascular access, but there are a number of intermediate sized, general purpose devices available. These devices have interchangeable probes to allow different uses, and hence can fulfill most of the requirements of the intensive care physician. It is not necessary to have large, state-of-the-art scanners often found in radiology departments; indeed, more expensive scanners may electronically filter some of the artifact that is necessary for diagnosis of certain pulmonary conditions.

Detailed visualization of vascular structures and the chest wall requires linear probes with higher frequency (4–10 MHz), whereas scanning the lung parenchyma and abdomen requires greater penetration and hence a lower frequency (2–4 MHz). Deeper scanning is often better performed with a curvilinear or phased array probe which will provide better contact and a larger field of view.

For sterile procedures there are a range of sheaths available to isolate the probe. Many devices have needle guides that can be clipped on to the probe head. Needle guides can display the projected trajectory of an attached needle on the screen; however, this is not always accurate as needles can deflect when pressure is applied, moving out of the field of view. We would recommend a freehand technique with careful visualization of the needle tip, rather than reliance on guides, although they are useful for

Ultrasound in Anesthetic Practice, ed. Graham Arthurs and Barry Nicholls. Published by Cambridge University Press.
© Cambridge University Press 2009.

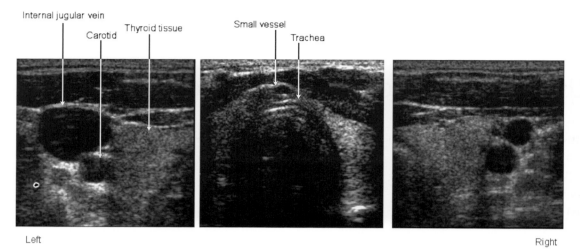

Figure 6.1   Anterior neck anatomy. Composite of three images of one of the authors' necks. The trachea in the central image is flanked by images of vessels on the left and right. It is worth noting the difference in size of the left and right internal jugular veins, making the left-sided vessel a potentially better target. The internal jugular vein also lies anterior to the carotid sheath on both sides, rendering the transfixion of the vessel potentially hazardous. Ultrasound can be used to guide the needle from medial to lateral in order to avoid the artery. There is also a small vessel lying anterior to the trachea, which may be of relevance to tracheotomy.

teaching. It is also worth noting that these guides are usually single-use only and are therefore expensive for routine use.

Ultrasound anatomy

Understanding of the underlying anatomy is vital to the success of any ultrasound-guided procedure. It is also important to appreciate the differing ultrasound appearances of air, fluid and solid tissue. Most ICU ultrasound is limited to the neck (for vascular access and tracheostomy), the chest (for pleural drainage and diagnosis of parenchymal pathology), and the abdomen (usually restricted to drainage procedures). We present a brief review of the anatomy of these areas which will illustrate the relevant ultrasonic appearances.

Scanning can take place in either the longitudinal or transverse plane in relation to the underlying structure. In the longitudinal plane an underlying vessel will appear long and thin; the transverse plane produces a rounded cross-sectional view of the vessel.

Ultrasound anatomy 1 – the anterior neck and subclavian region

The ability to correctly distinguish arteries, veins and air-filled structures (trachea and lung apex) from the surrounding soft tissues is the key to successful ultrasound-guided procedures in the neck. Liquid is anechoic (does not reflect ultrasound) and appears black. Air-filled structures reflect ultrasound and hence little can be seen beyond the air–tissue interface. Soft tissue transmits ultrasound to a greater or lesser extent depending on its relative density and water content.

Arteries and veins both appear black. Differentiation of the two is based on pulsatility, and collapsibility. Arteries are pulsatile, the appearance of which is often enhanced by gentle pressure with the ultrasound probe, which will also demonstrate the fact that they do not collapse easily. Veins are thin-walled and collapse under minimal pressure. They may be seen to alter dimensions with the respiratory cycle, but venous pulsations are not usually seen.

The position of the internal jugular vein in relation to the carotid artery is variable, and this highlights one of the great advantages of ultrasound. The artery may lie laterally to the vein, and landmark-based techniques may then fail. The ability to correctly differentiate arteries and veins, whatever their position, will help to avoid potentially disastrous arterial puncture (Figure 6.1 and video 6.2, on DVD, Anterior neck anatomy).

Ultrasound-guided subclavian access is possible, but usually requires a more lateral approach than is traditionally taught. The clavicle completely reflects ultrasound, producing an acoustic shadow that obliterates the subclavian vein underlying it. Moving the probe laterally will demonstrate the subclavian vessels as they become the axillary artery and vein (between the outer border of teres major and the lateral border of the first rib). In this position the chest wall is falling away inferiorly and posteriorly, and the artery and vein are lying further apart, reducing the risks of attempted cannulation even further [7, 8]. Supraclavicular approaches can also be used.

The trachea is easily located in the center of the anterior neck. The air–tissue interface on the inner surface of the trachea will reflect ultrasound, and generates artifacts (Figure 6.3, on DVD). The trachea then appears as a white walled structure, filled with black air with artifactual concentric rings within it. The tracheal rings can be differentiated in the tracheal wall. With experience it is possible to identify tracheal rings and the cricoid cartilage and use this information to guide percutaneous tracheostomy procedures [9]. Vessels in front of the trachea are easily visualized and avoided.

Ultrasound anatomy 2 – the pleura

The pleural space is relatively easy to visualize. Although the inferior pleural areas can be seen with a transabdominal approach (either through the liver or through the spleen), direct scanning through the chest wall is often better as this will

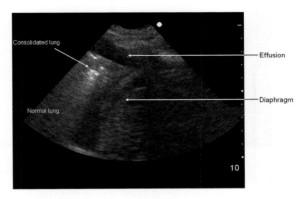

Figure 6.5 Pleural effusion. Pleural effusion with partially consolidated lung. This image was taken with the long axis lying in a caudal–cephalad orientation. The effusion separates the lung from the chest wall and the diaphragm, making it easy to differentiate the various structures. Normal lung is usually obscured by artifact generated at the pleural border.

usually be the approach needed for any proposed drainage procedure.

The parietal and visceral pleura are normally closely applied. The parietal pleura is static and appears as a distinct white line, whereas the visceral pleura moves with respiration and is less distinct. This moving pleural line has been termed the sliding lung sign. Introduction of fluid or air into the pleural space results in separation of the pleura, and this forms the basis of scanning prior to drainage procedures (Figure 6.4, on DVD).

Separation of the pleura by an area of anechoic fluid suggests pleural effusion (Figures 6.5 and 6.6, on DVD). If the effusion is large then it may be difficult to see the visceral pleura unless a probe with sufficient penetration is available. Pleural fluid is not always clear; cloudy fluid with visible particles floating within it suggests an exudate. Loculations can often be seen within the fluid, as can strands of fibrin. This is an important finding, as ultrasound-guided drainage will only usually enter a single locule, and whilst it is possible to make multiple needle passes into individual locules, this requires great skill and can be dangerous. If locules

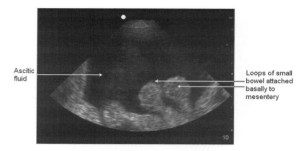

Ascitic fluid

Loops of small bowel attached basally to mesentery

10

Figure 6.7 Ascites. This image demonstrates the appearance of ascitic fluid. The fluid is anechoic and therefore appears black. Small bowel is seen rising from the bottom of the image. This image demonstrates a reasonably safe area to perform an ascitic tap as the fluid is deep, and the visceral structures are well away from the anterior peritoneum.

are detected then a traditional, open intercostal drain with a "finger sweep" may be more appropriate. Some patients will require formal surgical debridement.

Estimation of the volume of an effusion is possible and a number of methods have been suggested [10]. This information may guide decisions about whether to drain an effusion or not, but on ICU this decision is usually clinical, based on the difficulties in oxygenation and stage of illness. We would not routinely drain an effusion unless it was felt to have diagnostic importance or we felt that drainage would provide a significant benefit in gas exchange (greater than 1000 ml in an adult). An appropriate puncture site can be chosen by assessing depth of the effusion at the proposed site.

Identification of air in the pleural space is more difficult. Air does not transmit ultrasound and the operator must rely on the absence of the normal lung appearances.

Ultrasound anatomy 3 – the peritoneum

Identification of peritoneal collections follows a similar pattern to pleural collections. A detailed review of the abdominal anatomy as seen on ultrasound is clearly beyond the scope of this chapter; however, basic anatomical knowledge will help

the operator identify most major structures through their position and typical appearance.

Correct identification of fluid and the limitations of the space to be drained is again the key to successful drainage. Fluid will again appear black, viscera gray (Figures 6.7 and 6.8, on DVD). The position of the bowel is very variable as it moves freely within the fluid. It is important therefore to ensure that any proposed drainage site is free of viscera that could be damaged by a drainage procedure; gas-filled bowel will float, and hence positioning the patient may help.

Needle visualization

The ability to visualize the needle and accurately guide its movements are common to any needle-based technique using ultrasound guidance (Figure 6.9, on DVD).

Vascular access
Venous

Ultrasound-guided vascular access has become part of established practice in many UK ICUs. Guidelines from the National Institute for Clinical Excellence [11] have suggested routine use of ultrasound for all internal jugular lines, but there is also a reasonable body of evidence supporting the use of ultrasound for other sites of access [12]. The benefits of ultrasound are measured in terms of reduced complications, shorter procedure times and increased first puncture rates. Analysis also suggests that ultrasound-guided access produces an overall cost benefit [13, 14]. A recent randomized study of 900 critical care patients demonstrated clear benefit for ultrasound (US) in terms or procedural complications (Figure 6.10) and a trend towards a lower risk of catheter-related sepsis.

Two approaches can be taken.

(1) Preliminary scanning with identification of underlying vessels to confirm the position of the required patent vessel in relation to surface landmarks, then a blind procedure.

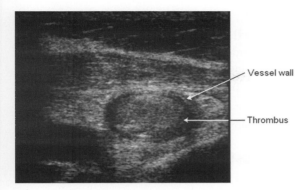

Figure 6.10 Thrombosed vessel. This image shows an occlusive thrombus in the lumen of the subclavian vein. The thrombus has a similar echogenicity to soft tissue and is not compressible. The vessel is clearly not suitable for cannulation. The chest wall can be seen in the lower right-hand corner of the image.

(2) Direct ultrasound guidance of the needle throughout the procedure.

The second option is intuitively safer, as it controls for any patient movement and allows adjustment of trajectory as the tissues are distorted by the needle. Puncture of deeper vessels (such as the axillary vein) require direct ultrasound guidance as the vessel position is not easy to relate to surface structures.

Whichever method is chosen, it is important to identify a reasonably straight length of vein that can be clearly visualized and has no overlying structures than to attempt puncture of a vessel in a traditional position that cannot be seen clearly with ultrasound. After insertion the guide-wire and catheter can be seen to be within the vessel lumen.

Arterial

Ultrasound has also been used to direct arterial cannulation. Puncture of the radial artery is often not difficult, and the complications related to not hitting the vessel are minimal (compared to the consequences of carotid puncture or damage to the trachea or pleura in the neck). However, ultrasound has been shown to improve the success rate for first time puncture and reduces the time taken for these procedures [15]. We do not use ultrasound for routine arterial cannulation when a strong distinct pulse is palpable, but increasingly we are using ultrasound to detect the radial artery in a more proximal position in the arm when the usual points in the wrist have been used and no pulse is palpable. This technique is also of value in the obese, edematous and severely shocked patients.

The position of the artery between the wrist and the ante-cubital fossa is not easy to predict, and hence we recommend tracing distally from the brachial pulsation, or its anticipated position medial to the biceps tendon insertion. In this way it is usually possible to identify a good position for cannulation in the mid forearm (Figure 6.11, on DVD). The femoral artery is easily visualized with ultrasound allowing accurate placement of the needle in the common rather than superficial femoral artery and the avoidance, where possible, of significantly diseased arteries (Figure 6.12, on DVD).

Drainage procedures

Insertion of drains into pleural, peritoneal and other fluid collections is a standard procedure on the ICU. These procedures have traditionally been guided by plain radiographs and clinical assessment. CT is the gold standard for diagnosis and guidance of drainage in most situations, but exposes the patient to the risk of intra-hospital transfer and is expensive and time-consuming. Ultrasound provides a viable alternative to CT in most instances, allowing diagnosis and drainage at the bedside [16] and has been shown to be safe [17–19] and to improve first time aspiration of the effusion to be drained.

There are essentially two approaches to a drainage procedure:

(1) The area can be scanned, the target identified and the area marked. The procedure can then be performed without direct guidance. This procedure is safe if the patient does not move

between scanning and needle insertion, and the target is not close to vital structures that could be hit if the needle is not inserted exactly along the line of the previous scan.

(2) The area is scanned, the target identified and the drainage performed all under direct guidance with visualization of the needle at all times.

Although the technique of drain insertion is similar for all sites, understanding the anatomical appearances is important to ensure safe siting of any drain.

Drainage technique

There are a number of different drainage kits available commercially. Most of these employ a Seldinger guide-wire technique which will be familiar to most anesthetists. There are differences between the kits in terms of shape and design of drain, but these are often not important. Needle design also varies, the most important difference is that some kits come with a bevelled cutting needle, and some with a Huber tipped needle. It is important to recognize the difference between the two. The cutting needle is more prone to damaging viscera with its sharp tip, the Huber tipped needle is less likely to cut into viscera, but requires more force to advance through the tissues. The Huber tipped needle is ideal for pleural drainage as the ribs will prevent deformation of the chest wall as the needle is advanced.

Drainage procedures should be performed with full sterile technique, with all appropriate resuscitative equipment and an assistant available at all times. There should be adequate light, but this should be adjustable as the ultrasound screen may not be easily viewable in bright light.

The patient should be positioned to allow dependent pooling of any fluid, but also adequate access to the proposed drainage site. Traditionally pleural drainage is best performed sitting with the arm raised above the head; this may not be practical in the ICU patient and hence positioning is usually a compromise between what is ideal and what is achievable. Remember that air-filled viscera (lung and bowel) will usually float and fluid will collect in a dependent manner.

The ultrasound device should be positioned so that it can be easily seen throughout the procedure and the operators gaze can move between the operative site and the screen without changing position.

Tracheostomy

Ultrasound has been shown to reduce the incidence of bleeding complications and improve correct positioning of the tracheostomy, and as such is recommended prior to percutaneous tracheostomy. Identification of vessels in the anterior neck informs decisions about the safety of a percutaneous approach and the need for surgical tracheostomy. Use of the ultrasound during the procedure can guide the operator away from vessels and into the trachea, whilst maintaining a bridge of tissue between the tracheostomy and any vascular structures [20–22]. Open dissection and exposure of these vessels requires ligation and division of the vessel, skills which are not common to all intensivists.

It is important to recognize that the vessels that are being looked for are often veins and hence will collapse under minimal pressure, especially in the head up position. Lay the patient flat or head down in order to obtain the best views. A Valsalva maneuvre may help open collapsed vessels.

Identification of the tracheal rings on ultrasound allows the operator to place the needle accurately, avoiding laryngeal structures and the risk of long-term stenosis that high tracheostomy generates. This may not be necessary if bronchoscopic guidance is to be used, but is often helpful in the obese where identification of surface landmarks is difficult.

Diagnostic scanning

As experience with ultrasound grows, intensivists are expanding the range of their scanning. Scanning

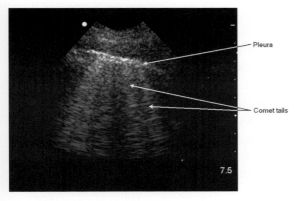

Figure 6.13 Comet tails in pulmonary edema. This image demonstrates the appearance of pulmonary edema. Four comet tails are seen in this image; they arise from the pleural border and spread to the edge of the image. The typical bright appearance of the pleura can also be seen.

Normal lung

Normal, well-aerated lung is difficult to see on ultrasound as the air-filled lung completely reflects ultrasound signals; however, as soon as liquid or solid matter becomes applied to the visceral pleura an "acoustic window" is opened and allows visualization of underlying structures [23]. The visceral pleura will be seen to slide against the parietal pleura with respiration. Beyond the visceral pleura, normal lung is identifiable by the lack of distinct detail; instead, there appear lines generated by reverberation artifact from the highly reflective lung chest wall interface. These lines repeat at regular intervals and are parallel and have been termed A-lines [24, 25].

Pulmonary edema

Detection of pulmonary edema relies on artifacts generated by interstitial fluid. This fluid generates a typical "comet tail" appearance of narrow lines spreading radially from the pleural surface (termed B-lines). These lines should be well defined and spread to the limit of the ultrasound devices depth of penetration. In order to be pathological, it is necessary for there to be multiple (at least three) comet tails present in a single intercostal window, and that these are either disseminated, or confined to the lateral chest wall. Small comet tails are normal in the dependent lung [26]. The presence of comet tails has been used to successfully differentiate between COPD and pulmonary edema [27] and has been shown to correlate well with measurements of extravascular lung water from PICCO, and a raised wedge pressure from pulmonary artery (PA) catheters [28].

Pneumothorax

Pneumothorax is diagnosed by the lack of the normal appearance of the pleura sliding against one another and the absence of the pattern of artifact seen in normal lung. In M-mode ultrasound the

the abdomen is difficult due to the number of different organs and their range of normal and pathological appearance. Beyond the identification of ascitic collections, we currently leave abdominal scanning to qualified radiologists and radiographers. Scanning the chest is somewhat simpler with echocardiography a separate subject (see Chapter 3). Ultrasound can be used to diagnose a number of pulmonary conditions including pulmonary edema (Figure 6.13), pneumothorax, atelectasis, consolidation and even pulmonary embolism, often with greater sensitivity than plain radiograph and without recourse to CT scanning. We will briefly review the appearances of normal lung and the changes that occur in disease.

Although it is possible to localize a scan to areas of interest seen on radiograph it is important to use a systematic approach so that all areas of the lung have been visualized and no pathology is missed. There are various methods of doing this, but all essentially involve dividing the surface of the thorax into discrete zones and then systematically scanning each area; it is important not to neglect the posterior surface of the lung.

normal granular appearance of the lung is replaced by a linear pattern. Small pneumothoraces, not visible on plain radiograph, can be detected in this manner [24].

Consolidation

Consolidation is visible only when it extends to the lung edge. Interposition of air between the probe and the pathology will generate artifact as seen in normal lung. Consolidated lung looks dense and bronchograms can be seen. This appearance is often termed hepatization, as the solid lung has a similar appearance to liver.

Pulmonary embolism (PE)

Diagnosis of PE with ultrasound relies on the detection of wedge-shaped areas of infarction visible arising from the pleural line, with the apex of the wedge pointing towards the mediastinum. The presence of two or more of these lesions, combined with a positive history and no other relevant chest findings (e.g. consolidation), has been shown to be a reasonable alternative to CT of the pulmonary arteries [29]. It seems unlikely that ultrasound will replace CT for the diagnosis of PE, but is a useful alternative when CT is not available, or the patient is too ill to transfer.

Conclusions

Ultrasound is an emerging speciality on ICU, and is likely to become more prevalent in the future as experience grows. Ultrasound is cost-effective, non-invasive and is free of the complications of radiation exposure and transfer that are present with other imaging modalities. We would encourage anesthetists and intensivists to familiarize themselves with the appearance of normal lung and pleural and peritoneal pathology by regular scanning of ICU patients and comparison of their findings with plain radiographs and CT. Involvement of the radiology department is recommended when diagnosis is not clear.

REFERENCES

1. Kannan S. Another use for ultrasound in the ICU. *Anaesthesia* 2005;60(9):944.
2. Dorffner R, Eibenberger K, Youssefzadeh S, *et al*. The value of sonography in the intensive care unit for the diagnosis of diaphragmatic paralysis. *RöFo: Fortschritte auf dem Gebiete der Röntgenstrahlen und der Nuklearmedizin* 1998;169(3):274–7.
3. Civardi G, Di Candio G, Giorgi A, *et al*. Ultrasound guided percutaneous drainage of abdominal abscesses in the hands of the clinician: a multicenter Italian study. *European Journal of Ultrasound: Official Journal of the European Federation of Societies for Ultrasound in Medicine and Biology* 1998;8(2):91–9.
4. Ebaugh JL, Chiou AC, Morasch MD, *et al*. Bedside vena cava filter placement guided with intravascular ultrasound. *Journal of Vascular Surgery: Official Publication of the Society for Vascular Surgery (and) International Society for Cardiovascular Surgery North American Chapter* 2001;34(1):21–6.
5. Bouch DC, AP Hall. Ultrasound diagnosis of a false radial artery aneurysm in ICU. *Anaesthesia* 2006;61(10):1018.
6. Bodenham AR. Editorial II: Ultrasound imaging by anaesthetists: training and accreditation issues. *British Journal of Anaesthesia* 2006;96(4):414–7.
7. Galloway S, Bodenham A. Ultrasound imaging of the axillary vein – anatomical basis for central venous access. *British Journal of Anaesthesia* 2003;90(5):589–95.
8. Sharma A, Bodenham AR, Mallick A. Ultrasound-guided infraclavicular axillary vein cannulation for central venous access. *British Journal of Anaesthesia* 2004;93(2):188–92.
9. Sustic A, Kovac D, Zgaljardic Z, *et al*. Ultrasound-guided percutaneous dilatational tracheostomy: a safe method to avoid cranial misplacement of the tracheostomy tube.

Intensive Care Medicine 2000;26(9):1379–81.

10. Vignon P, Chastagner C, Berkane V, *et al.* Quantitative assessment of pleural effusion in critically ill patients by means of ultrasonography. *Critical Care Medicine* 2005;33(8):1757–63.

11. Guidance on the use of ultrasound locating devices for central venous catheters (NICE technology appraisal, No. 49.) London: NICE. 2002. www.nice.org.uk.

12. Hind D, Calvert N, McWilliams R, *et al.* Ultrasonic locating devices for central venous cannulation: meta-analysis. *British Medical Journal (Clinical Research Edition)* 2003; 327(7411):361.

13. Calvert N, Hind D, McWilliams R, *et al.* Ultrasound for central venous cannulation: economic evaluation of cost-effectiveness. *Anaesthesia* 2004;59(11):1116–20.

14. Calvert N, Hind D, McWilliams R, *et al.* The effectiveness and cost-effectiveness of ultrasound locating devices for central venous access: a systematic review and economic evaluation. *Health Technology Assessment (Winchester England)* 2003;7(12):1–84.

15. Levin PD, Sheinin O, Gozal Y. Use of ultrasound guidance in the insertion of radial artery catheters. *Critical Care Medicine* 2003; 31(2):481–4.

16. van Sonnenberg E, Wiltich GR, Goodare BW, Znisschenberg JB. Percutaneous drainage of thoracic collections. *Journal of Thoracic Imaging* 1998;13(2):74–82.

17. Singh H. One more use of ultrasound in ICU. *Anaesthesia* 2006;61(4):407.

18. Mayo PH, Golt Z, Tafreshi MI, Doelken P. Safety of ultrasound-guided thoracocentesis in patients receiving mechanical ventilation. *Chest* 2004;125(3):1059–62.

19. Jones P.W, Moyers JP, Rogers JT, *et al.* Ultrasound-guided thoracocentesis: is it a safer method? *Chest* 2003;123(2):418–23.

20. Muhammad JK, Patton DW, Evans RM, Major E. Percutaneous dilatational tracheostomy under ultrasound guidance. *The British Journal of Oral & Maxillofacial Surgery* 1999;37(4): 309–11.

21. Kollig E, Heydenreich U, Roetman B. Ultrasound and bronchoscopic controlled percutaneous tracheostomy on trauma ICU. *Injury* 2000;31(9):663–8.

22. Hatfield A, Bodenham A. Portable ultrasonic scanning of the anterior neck before percutaneous dilatational tracheostomy. *Anaesthesia* 1999;54(7):660–3.

23. Beaulieu Y, Marik PE. Bedside ultrasonography in the ICU: part 2. *Chest* 2005;128(3):1766–81.

24. Lichtenstein DA, Mezière G, Lascals N, *et al.* Ultrasound diagnosis of occult pneumothorax. *Critical Care Medicine* 2005;33(6):1231–8.

25. Diacon AH, Theron J, Bolliger CT. Transthoracic ultrasound for the pulmonologist. *Current Opinion in Pulmonary Medicine* 2005;11(4):307–12.

26. Lichtenstein D, Meziere G, Biderman P, Gepner A. The comet-tail artefact. An ultrasound sign of alveolar-interstitial syndrome. *American Journal of Respiratory and Critical Care Medicine* 1997;156(5):1640–6.

27. Lichtenstein D, Mezière G. A lung ultrasound sign allowing bedside distinction between pulmonary edema and COPD: the comet-tail artefact. *Intensive Care Medicine* 1998;24(12): 1331–4.

28. Agricola E, Bore T, Oppizi M, *et al.* Ultrasound comet-tail images: a marker of pulmonary edema: a comparative study with wedge pressure and extravascular lung water. *Chest* 2005;127(5):1690–5.

29. Mathis G, Blank W, Reissig A, *et al.* Thoracic ultrasound for diagnosing pulmonary embolism: a prospective multicenter study of 352 patients. *Chest* 2005;128(3): 1531–8.

Chapter 7

Use of ultrasound in the traumatized patient and the acute abdomen

SAPNA PUPPALA, VISHWANATH ACHARYA, DAVID A. PARKER AND DENNIS LI. COCHLIN

Introduction

Ultrasound examination is quick, non-invasive and involves no ionizing radiation. Its portability enables the investigation to be performed at the bedside, making it an ideal tool in the investigation of acute abdominal conditions. In most of these clinical situations, ultrasound is used as the first line of imaging after radiological plain film. The recent advancement of FAST (Focused Abdominal Sonography for Trauma, also called Focused Assessment with Sonography for Trauma) has encouraged non-radiologists to use ultrasound for emergency assessment of blunt abdominal trauma [1]. Similarly, ultrasound can be used for quick bedside assessment of not only intra-abdominal free fluid but also pleural and pericardial fluid, aiding in speedy decision-making in intensive care units [2]. Ultrasound is operator-dependent and, in addition, bowel gas and patients' body habitus (more precisely fat content of the abdominal wall) pose further limitations to the diagnostic information obtainable from the examination. Because of these limitations, a comprehensive training in scanning techniques is essential before practicing and interpreting ultrasound in acute abdominal emergencies [3].

There are further practical considerations in acute abdominal sonography. Patient mobility may be restricted especially in trauma situations and in ITU. Time and space available for scanning may also be limited if the patient is clinically unstable. In cases of bowel perforation, the free intraperitoneal gas can obscure most of the underlying structures during an ultrasound scan.

Ultrasound anatomy of abdomen and pelvis

A sound knowledge of abdominal anatomy as well as sonographic features of normal structures are crucial in making a sonographic assessment of the acute abdomen. This section deals with the normal basic sonographic anatomy and techniques used in assessing the acute abdomen. Figure 7.1 (on DVD) is a schematic representation of the contents of the abdomen as seen in a frontal view. Ultrasound examination, however, is an assessment of these structures in cross-section in an axial, saggital or oblique plane as shown in Figures 7.2, 7.3 and 7.4. Patients can be turned around to obtain further views, as well as to assess mobile structures such as gallstones or to displace air or fluid.

Ultrasound in Anesthetic Practice, ed. Graham Arthurs and Barry Nicholls. Published by Cambridge University Press.
© Cambridge University Press 2009.

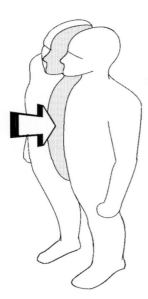

Figure 7.2 Sagittal view.

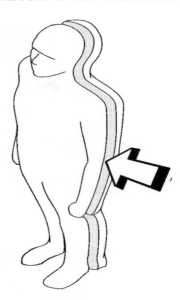

Figure 7.4 Coronal view.

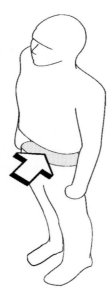

Figure 7.3 Axial view.

The ultrasound probe acts as both a transmitter and a receiver of sound waves. Depending on the organs they interact with in their path, the waves are either reflected (echoed) or allowed to pass through to varying degrees. Most solid organs such as the liver, spleen, kidneys and pancreas reflect (echo) the sound waves. Organs reflecting these

waves thus appear echogenic or bright. The higher the fat content the more echogenic the appearance. Structures containing fluid tend to allow the waves to pass through, such as a full bladder which therefore appears anechoic or black. Most pathology has an inflammatory component drawing fluid thus appearing less echogenic or hypo-echoic. Hemorrhage may appear bright when blood has coagulated, although fresh hyperacute blood is anechoic. After a short period of time, internal echoes develop, and later the hematoma liquefies and separates into serum and cellular component, making the serum appear anechoic. The anatomy of the important sites routinely scanned is shown in Figures 7.1 to 7.16. While scanning a patient, one has to bear in mind the clinical question which needs to be answered, and scanning should be directed towards the relevant specific organs. Important views used in acute assessment are described under individual sections.

(1) Morrison's pouch – Figures 7.5 and 7.6 (on DVD).

(2) Spleno-renal space – Figures 7.7 and 7.8 (on DVD).

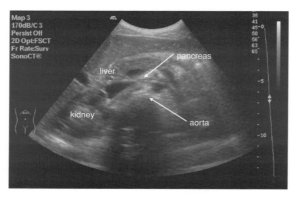

Figure 7.9 Axial view of midline structures of upper abdomen.

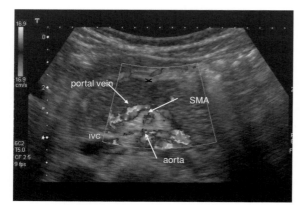

Figure 7.10 Deep sonography showing vascular anatomy of upper abdomen.

(3) Midline axial of upper abdomen with pancreas and aorta – Figures 7.9, 7.10 and 7.11 (on DVD).
(4) Midline aorta – Figure 7.12 (on DVD).
(5) Bladder axial – Figures 7.13 and 7.14 (both on DVD).
(6) Bladder sagittal and free fluid in pouch of Douglas – Figures 7.15 and 7.16 (both on DVD).

Ultrasound of abdominal trauma – FAST Scans

Traditional methods of assessment of blunt abdominal trauma include diagnostic peritoneal lavage and computed tomography (CT) of the abdomen.

Though US was used in the assessment of abdominal trauma, the concept of Focused Abdominal Sonography for Trauma (FAST) has been introduced in the last 10 years, initially in the United States. FAST is gaining increasing acceptance in Europe as a method of evaluation of blunt abdominal trauma. The main focus of the examination is detection of free fluid in the abdomen secondary to injury of the abdominal organs [4]. Clinically unstable patients involved in trauma in whom significant free fluid is detected on ultrasound are immediately taken for laparotomy without undergoing CT correlation. Solid intra-abdominal organs can also be imaged to locate the source of bleeding if time permits. Various studies have quoted sensitivities of 85–100% and specificities of 98–100% for the FAST technique [4]. Reported sensitivities for detecting solid organ trauma by ultrasound have been quoted at 41% [3, 4].

Technique

The technique for detection of free fluid involves scanning various areas of abdomen and pelvis systematically looking for anechoic (black) or hypoechoic free fluid. Even though various authors suggest different techniques, the overall aim is to cover all quadrants of the abdomen and pelvis while scanning. A 3.5 MHz curvilinear probe is the most suitable probe. An acceptable sequence would include examination of at least four regions, as shown in Figure 7.17.
(1) Right upper quadrant (hepato-renal pouch and peri-hepatic region).
(2) Epigastrium to look for pericardial effusions by placing the probe immediate to the right of the xiphisternum parallel to the left costal margin while focusing the ultrasound beam to the left and upwards to visualize the interface between the right ventricle and the pericardium.
(3) Left upper quadrant (peri-splenic area and spleno-renal region).
(4) Pelvis axial and longitudinal views.

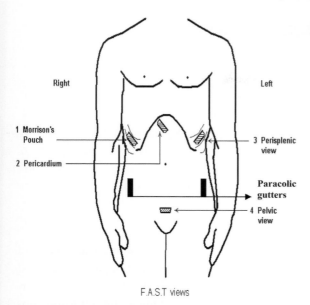

Figure 7.17 FAST technique.

FAST–4fs (technique)
Free fluid
Four quadrants and
  pericardium
Four solid organs if time
  permits
Forget not the fluid from
  pelvic wall fractures

FAST–5Ps (quadrants)
Perihepatic
Perisplenic
Pelvic
Pericardium
Paracolic gutters

Ideally the pelvis should be examined with a full bladder. If time and circumstances permit, evaluation of the solid organs (liver, spleen and both kidneys) may be undertaken to assess any injuries suggestive of source of bleeding.

Ultrasound findings in FAST

The cornerstone of FAST is the detection of free fluid. Free fluid is anechoic or homogeneously hypoechoic. However, in some cases it may have some internal echoes depending on the nature of the fluid and the time interval for blood to clot. Focal echogenic areas close to the site of injury may represent a hematoma. Free fluid usually has a triangular shape when it collects around bowel loops and a linear shape if between liver and kidney. Free fluid commonly accumulates in depen-

Table 7.1 Free fluid scoring system (Sirlin et al. [5])

No. of collections	Severity of injury (%)	Need for intervention (%)
0	1.4	0.4
1	59	13
2	85	36
3	83	63

The more the amount of fluid, the more the chance of injury and intervention needed.

dent peritoneal recesses such as the paracolic gutters and pelvis, and around the liver and spleen. Pericardial effusion is also seen as an anechoic collection in the pericardial space. Moderate amounts of fluid will be readily diagnosed by experienced operators, whilst smaller amounts are difficult to observe and interpret. Intra-abdominal free fluid collections have been graded by various authors and correlated to severity of injury and surgical intervention needed. Systems of free fluid scoring have also been published such as by Sirlin et al., where for every anatomic location where fluid was found, a point was given [5]. The total number of points correlated to the severity of injuries and the intervention needed as shown in Table 7.1 [5].

Other injuries

Solid organ injuries are usually seen as echogenic areas on US although specific features can be seen in some organs (Tables 7.2 and 7.3). Liver injury can manifest in various patterns.

Discrete or diffuse hyperechoic, discrete hypoechoic or echogenic clot or fluid may sometimes surround the liver. The most common pattern of splenic injury is a diffuse heterogeneous (mixed echogenic) appearance. Discrete hyperechoic or hypoechoic regions within the traumatized spleen may also be identified on US. A hyperechoic or hypoechoic rim or crescent, representing a clot, often surrounds the spleen (the peri-splenic subcapsular hematomas) [6]. Renal parenchymal

Table 7.2 Patterns of solid organ injury on ultrasound

Organ	Pattern	Nature
1. Liver	Hyperechoic – discrete or diffuse	Contusions
	Hypoechoic – discrete	Laceration
	Echogenic – discrete	Clot
	Peri-hepatic echogenic	Collection/hematoma
2. Spleen	Heterogenous – diffuse	Contusions
	Hyperechoic – discrete	Blood in laceration
	Hypoechoic – discrete	Laceration
	Echogenic or hypoechoic subcapsular	Peri-splenic hematoma
3. Kidneys	Mixed echogenic	Laceration
	Disorganized with loss of reniform shape	Severe lacerations

Table 7.3 Algorithmic approach to FAST scanning a trauma patient

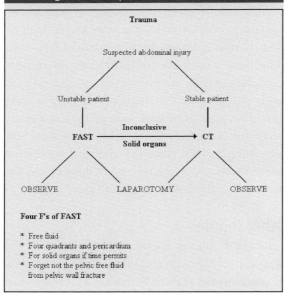

injuries are more difficult to detect on ultrasound. Severe renal lacerations are seen as mixed echogenic areas within the renal fossa and a completely disorganized appearance may be present with loss of reniform shape.

Case scenario 1

A 38-year-old builder was involved in a fall from a height of approximately 10 feet and landed on his left side. He sustained minor bruising over the left chest wall and was brought to the accident and emergency department by ambulance. On clinical examination, he was noticed to have diffuse tenderness over the upper abdomen and left lower thorax. Vital signs were as follows: Pulse110/min, BP 90/64, temperature 36.6 °C. An emergency ultrasound of the abdomen was carried out and following are some of the images. Figures 7.18 and 7.19 (both on DVD) show free fluid between the spleen and the left kidney; Figure 7.20 (on DVD) shows a subcapsular splenic hematoma; Figure 7.21 (on DVD) shows free fluid in the pouch of Douglas; Figure 7.22 (on DVD) shows free fluid in Morrison's space, and Figures 7.23 and 7.24 show different types of liver injury.

Limitations of FAST

In spite of the high sensitivity and specificity of FAST, operators need to be aware of potential pitfalls of this technique [6]. Free fluid in the pelvis could be missed if the bladder is not full and this could result in a false negative result. Therefore, whenever possible, a full bladder technique should be employed while scanning the pelvis for free fluid. As trauma patients tend to be catheterized in order to monitor output, the aim should be to either scan before catheterization or to clamp the catheter if possible. In women of reproductive age, a small amount of physiological free fluid can be seen in

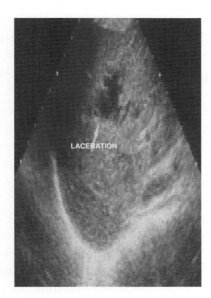

Figure 7.23 RUQ view showing laceration of the liver.

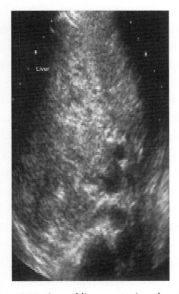

Figure 7.24 RUQ view of liver contusion showing a diffuse heterogeneous change.

the pouch of Douglas. It is then important to search for fluid in other sites to confirm the nature of fluid in the pouch of Douglas. Furthermore, FAST scans can miss important organ injuries requiring urgent surgical intervention. Patients on peritoneal dialysis or those with known ascites may pose a dilemma,

as there is pre-existing fluid in the pelvis. Dilated fluid filled loops of bowel can be misinterpreted as fluid collections. One must observe for peristalsis and also note the shape of bowel, which is more rounded and defined. Echogenic collections can be overlooked if one is not specifically looking for them. Ultrasound sensitivity for detection of free fluid associated with bowel or mesenteric injury is less than 50%, and US may not directly show any of the injuries to the bowel or mesentery [6]. In addition, ultrasound is unable to detect some significant internal injuries, such as diaphragmatic ruptures, vascular, pancreatic and adrenal injuries [6]. A contrast-enhanced CT scan of the abdomen and pelvis should be performed in a hemodynamically stable patient with blunt abdominal trauma in whom ultrasound suggests intra-abdominal injury [6]. Ultrasound has a proven value in the initial assessment of blunt abdominal trauma and can help in making life-saving clinical decisions in this group of patients. It is an important clinical tool in triaging acute blunt abdominal trauma patients in the accident and emergency department. A good hands-on training in scanning techniques as well as awareness of limitations of the technique is essential for professionals undertaking the examinations in the accident and emergency department [7]. Figure 7.25 (on DVD) shows a scan from a patient on dialysis with known abdominal trauma. It is difficult here to state the nature of the free fluid.

Abdominal emergencies

The acute abdomen can pose a diagnostic dilemma in clinical practice, and ultrasound over the last two to three decades has been a very important tool in clinical diagnosis. In this chapter we have tried to deal with a few of the common acute abdominal conditions such as abdominal aortic aneurysms, acute appendicitis, acute cholecystitis, acute urinary retention, and intra-abdominal collections such as diverticular abscesses and psuedocyst. The scanning technique involves meticulous assessment of all nine quadrants of the abdomen. Even though this could be performed in any order, it is advisable to scan the affected and usually the most tender area of the abdomen towards the end. In most cases a curvilinear 3.5 MHz probe is appropriate for scanning the abdomen. However, in cases of suspected acute appendicitis, a 5 MHz linear probe should also be used to assess the right iliac fossa, especially in thin patients using a graded compression technique [8]. As discussed before, most acute inflammatory conditions draw fluid into the organ, its wall or the vicinity. This acts as an indirect tool to guide the imaging. In women of reproductive age group, the presence of a tiny amount of fluid in the pouch of Douglas can be a normal variant, as shown in Figure 7.15 (on DVD).

Abdominal aortic aneurysm

Abdominal aortic aneurysms (AAA) are dilatations of the aorta which routinely are fusiform but can be saccular. They increase in incidence with age, and elderly men are at most risk. One may also come across an AAA while scanning the abdomen of patients with acute abdomen of unclear etiology in the accident and emergency department or encounter AAA while scanning a hypotensive patient in ITU. Abdominal aortic aneurysms may or may not be symptomatic when detected, but if they are, abdominal or back pain is the commonest presenting symptom. A leaking aneurysm is a surgical emergency and only 50% of patients make it to the accident and emergency department, where they present with pain with or without hypotension. In patients with a known history of aneurysm, making the diagnosis of a possible leak is straightforward, but those patients unaware of the condition need imaging to confirm or refute the presence of an AAA. In the presence of a known aneurysm, a contrast-enhanced CT scan is the investigation of choice provided the patient is hemodynamically

stable. Patients who are hemodynamically unstable in whom a rupture of an abdominal aneurysm has been suspected need urgent surgery rather than any form of imaging. Ultrasound may be helpful in patients with no known aneurysm and a vague clinical picture to confirm or exclude an aneurysm. Ultrasound is not reliable in detecting a leak, as some leaking aneurysms may cause a retroperitoneal hematoma which is not always appreciated at ultrasound, and a CT is more reliable here.

Technique

A curvilinear 3.5 MHz transducer is used to scan the midline starting from epigastrium in both longitudinal and transverse planes. Bowel gas shadows may obscure the abdominal aorta and applying gentle pressure and angling the transducer may help. An oblique or decubitus position or scanning on either side of the spine may help. An erect scan, although not practical in an acute situation, may also be used to displace the gas-filled bowel loop [9]. The normal maximal cross-sectional diameter of the aorta should not exceed 3 cm at any level. While assessing the abdominal aortic aneurysm, not only its size but also its location with respect to the renal arteries (infrarenal or suprarenal) and extent into the iliacs should be noted. The greater the diameter, the higher the risk of aneurysm rupture. Surgery is generally recommended when an aortic aneurysm exceeds 5.5 cm [10] (Tables 7.4a and 7.4b).

Figure 7.26 (on DVD) is of a 62-year-old male who was brought in with vague abdominal pain and became hypotensive in the accident and emergency department. ECG showed minor ST elevation. A US scan (USS) was done to confirm the presence of an AAA prior to theater.

Acute cholecystitis

Acute cholecystitis is inflammation of the gall bladder which commonly occurs due to obstruction by of the cystic duct by gallstones. Occasionally

Table 7.4a Algorithmic approach to imaging a leaking abdominal aortic aneurysm

- 3.5 MHz curvilinear probe
- Upper abdomen axial and sagittal views
- Anechoic fusiform or saccular structure
- Flow on Doppler
- Can have thrombus in the wall
- Measure outer wall to outer wall including thrombus (normal <3 cm)
- Assess the pelvis for free fluid which suggests a possible leak
- CT is superior to asses a leak if patient stable
- If patient unstable, USS used only to confirm AAA if needed (clinical ambiguity) prior to theater

Table 7.5 Checklist for ultrasound of acute cholecystitis

- RUQ examination
- 3.5 MHz curvilinear probe
- Gall bladder wall thickness >3 mm
- Fluid around the GB wall
- Gallstones (confirm in left lateral position)
- Positive sonographic Murphy's sign
- Doppler shows increased flow
- In ITU patients on TPN can have gall bladder abnormalities

Table 7.4b Algorithmic approach to imaging a leaking abdominal aortic aneurysm

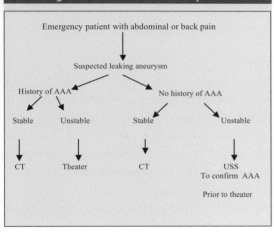

cholecystitis may occur in the absence of gallstones (acalculous cholecystitis). Patients present with acute pain in the right upper quadrant. On clinical examination, Murphy's sign is positive and inflammatory markers may be raised (Table 7.5).

Technique

A curvilinear 3.5 MHz probe is used to scan the right upper quadrant in both longitudinal and transverse planes. Depending on the location of the gall bladder in the abdomen, the right lower intercostal area may have to be used to access the gall blad-

der. Acute cholecystitis has a combination of specific sonographic findings which help in making an accurate diagnosis of the condition. The gall bladder wall is uniformly thickened due to acute inflammation (normal wall thickness is less than 3 mm). There may also be echo-poor areas in the gall bladder wall due to edema. There is usually a small hypoechoic rim of free fluid around the gall bladder. Doppler ultrasound is useful in that it usually shows increased blood flow around the inflamed gall bladder. One or more gallstones may be visible too, suggesting a diagnosis of acute calculous cholecystitis. A gallstone is visible as a bright, echogenic structure within the gall bladder lumen accompanied by a posterior acoustic shadowing. Another important indicator of the diagnosis of acute cholecystitis is the fact that gently pressing the ultrasound probe over the gall bladder point elicits pains (Murphy's equivalent). A combination of the above-mentioned findings supports the diagnosis of cholecystitis [11, 12]. A common pitfall is the prevalence of gall bladder abnormalities in ITU patients that are not due to cholecystitis making the diagnosis of acalculous cholecystitis even more difficult. In a study by Boland *et al.* [13], sludge, distention, wall thickening, and wall lucencies and pericholecystic fluid was observed in varying numbers in 44 of the 136 patients who underwent abdominal sonography in the ITU for suspected gall bladder pathology.

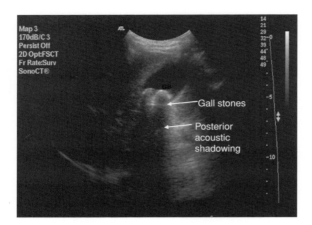

Figure 7.29 RUQ view showing gallstones in a normal-looking gall bladder.

Figure 7.27 (on DVD) shows a normal gall bladder; Figure 7.28 (on DVD) is from a 40-year-old, overweight, mother of two children presented to the emergency unit with pain in the right upper quadrant. Inflammatory markers were raised. US revealed a thick-walled inflamed gall bladder with stones; Figure 7.29 shows a gall bladder containing gallstones with characteristic posterior acoustic shadowing; Figure 7.30 (on DVD) shows another form of cholecystitis – emphysematous; Figure 7.31 (on DVD) is a gall bladder in an ITU patient on TPN showing echogenic bile but no inflammation in the wall.

Acute pancreatitis

This is a clinical and laboratory diagnosis and imaging features may not be apparent until 24–48 h after onset. A USS, however, can confirm the presence of gallstones and stones in the common bile duct with dilated biliary system. Initially the pancreas can have a spectrum of appearances from normal to edematous hypoechoic pattern. Free fluid can be seen in the region. In acute severe pancreatitis, more destruction of pancreas and collections can be seen. Focal pancreatitis is observed as hypoechoic foci in the pancreas which can be difficult to distinguish from a focal hypoechoic mass such as carcinoma.

Clinical correlation again is a useful tool with repeat scanning to assess resolution is a must. Pseudocyst is discussed under collections.

Acute appendicitis

Acute appendicitis is a common clinical condition presenting to accident and emergency department. The condition presents as acute abdominal pain, which begins in the periumbilical region and later localizes to the right iliac fossa. It may be associated with vomiting and pyrexia. Classically there is tenderness at McBurney's point. Ultrasound can be used to confirm the clinical diagnosis especially in clinically equivocal cases. In women, USS help to exclude pelvic inflammatory disease and tubo-ovarian causes of pain in the lower abdomen. However, one must remember that a negative scan does not exclude acute appendicitis.

Technique

A 5 MHz linear probe is used to scan the right lower abdomen. A graded compression method is used [8]. A normal appendix is difficult to visualize on ultrasound, but an inflamed thickened appendix can be seen. A gentle graded compression is applied over the region of appendix, which helps to establish diagnosis, as well as displace the bowel loops overlying the appendix. The loops of bowel and a normal appendix if visualized can be easily compressed as compared to an inflamed loop and appendix which cannot be compressed. Care should be taken while applying compression as this can cause discomfort to the patient. An inflamed appendix is enlarged and swollen and has a cross-sectional diameter of more than 6 mm. A small amount of free fluid may be present around an acutely inflamed appendix. However, a larger fluid collection around an inflamed appendix can suggests a perforated appendix with local peritonitis. An appendicolith may also be visible, and is seen as a hyperechoic structure with some posterior acoustic shadowing. With a suggestive clinical history, an

Table 7.6 Checklist for ultrasound of acute appendicitis

- 5 MHz linear probe
- RIF region
- Graded compression technique
- Thickened appendix of >6 mm
- Periappendicular free fluid
- Echogenic appendicolith with shadowing
- **Negative scan does not exclude appendicitis**
- Always scan the other quadrants of abdomen first. Using 3.5 MHz curvilinear probe

ill-defined hypo- or mixed-echogenic mass seen in the right iliac fossa, even when the appendix cannot be delineated, indicates a possible appendicular abscess. We would like to reiterate again that false negative scans are common, and the decision to operate is based on clinical judgment [14, 15] (Table 7.6).

Differential diagnosis

An important differential diagnosis to consider in young patients with right iliac fossa (RIF) pain is *Crohn's disease*. This has a predilection for terminal ileum but can affect the whole of the gastrointestinal tract. At ultrasound there is usually inflammation in the terminal ileum with thickening of the bowel wall and lack of peristalsis. A small amount of free fluid may be seen, and if advanced then an abscess or collection can be observed in the RIF. These features mimic appendicitis and make the diagnosis difficult. The key is proper clinical history and examination. The presence of a thickened inflamed appendix is more conclusive of appendicitis than of Crohn's. The remaining features, however, can exist in both conditions.

In women of child-bearing age, *ovarian cyst and torsions* are seen. The clinical features can resemble acute appendicitis but the laboratory results are not supportive. *Pelvic inflammatory disease*, however, can present as acute appendicitis with corresponding raised inflammatory markers. Associated vaginal discharge is an additional symptom if elicited. Vaginal examination, although not performed regularly in this day and age, helps in eliciting pelvic tenderness and assessing the pouch of Douglas. An ultrasound is therefore useful to differentiate the presence of an ovarian cyst and pelvic inflammatory disease (Figure 7.33 (on DVD)) from appendicitis.

A 20-year-old female patient presented with right iliac fossa and pelvic pain. She had inconclusive clinical signs and inflammatory markers were marginally raised. An US scan was performed that showed the hypoechoic tubular structure of the thickened inflamed appendix (Figure 7.32, on DVD).

Mesenteric ischemia

Patients in intensive care units are prone to mesenteric ischemia either from pre-existing atrial fibrillation or cardiovascular compromise and/or the use of ionotropes. An acidotic patient with distending abdomen and ileus is suspected of having mesenteric ischemia. Its early diagnosis has a bearing on the management of the patient in the form of surgery. Ultrasound can be used, but is not fully diagnostic. Inflamed thickened loops of distended bowel are non-specific features. The presence of echogenic air in its wall is more diagnostic. There may be associated free fluid. A more contributory finding is the presence of air seen as echogenic bright areas in the main portal veins, its branches in the liver and in the superior mesenteric vein. This suggests mucosal disruption of bowel with intraluminal air entering the venous circulation to reach the veins in the liver. An important differential is air in the biliary tree, which is commonly seen after ERCP and spincterotomy. Biliary air is confined to the periportal area as compared to portal air, which is distributed all over as a starry sky appearance. Figure 7.34 (on DVD) shows air in the portal vein – mesenteric ischemia.

Table 7.7 Checklist for ultrasound of acute retention

- 3.5 MHz curvilinear probe
- Axial and longitudinal views of pelvis
- Anechoic cystic structure suggests bladder
- Assess kidneys for hydronephrosis
- If bladder empty, consider anuria from prerenal, renal or post-renal causes such as bilateral ureteric obstruction

Acute retention

In patients with anuria, distinguishing between urinary retention and other causes of poor urine output can be achieved with a simple scan of the urinary bladder.

Technique

A 3.5 MHz curvilinear probe is used to examine the pelvis both axially and longitudinally with a full sweep from side to side as well as top to bottom until the pubic bone is seen. The presence of a large anechoic pear-shaped structure in longitudinal view and a square or rectangle on axial view confirms the presence of a full bladder and acute retention, which can be relieved easily by catheterization. The prostate, which may be visibly enlarged, is a common underlying cause of urinary retention. Hydronephrosis may complicate chronic urinary retention, but when accompanying an empty bladder implies ureteric obstruction. In women, caution has to be exercised as rarely a large simple ovarian cyst may be mistaken for bladder (Table 7.7).

A 60-year-old male patient presented to the accident and emergency department with inability to pass urine (Figure 7.35, on DVD). An emergency US scan performed shows an anechoic distended bladder. This was catheterized immediately and the patient was relieved of his symptoms. Figure 7.36 (on DVD) shows hydronephrosis in a patient presenting with right-sided renal colic.

Intra-abdominal collections

Intra-abdominal collections usually result from infections, inflammations, trauma, bleeding, postoperative and leak from intra-abdominal organs, such as a bowel, biliary or urinary leak, again usually due to intraoperative damage. The most commonly encountered collections are post-operative, due to perforations, or secondary to pancreatitis. Collections are anechoic (black) if the fluid is simple, but varying degrees of echogenicity may be seen depending on complications such as infections or bleeding [16, 17]. Ultrasound is used not only to diagnose but to perform ultrasound-guided aspirations or drainages of these collections. CT guidance is also used to drain collections; more so when the presence of air in the collection makes US scan-guided procedure difficult or impossible [18]. The management of pancreatic pseudocyst varies on the patient's clinical condition and the nature of the contents of the cyst. If asymptomatic, then they are left to resolve on their own. If symptomatic and causing obstruction, they may be drained either percutaneously, with endoluminal ultrasound or surgically. These should, however, be performed by trained experts.

Figure 7.37: US scan of a 40-year-old patient with acute on chronic pancreatitis secondary to alcohol

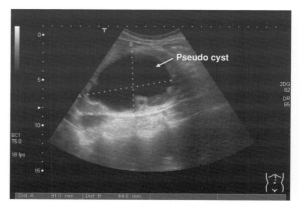

Figure 7.37 Pseudocyst in a patient known to have chronic pancreatitis.

shows an anechoic cyst with a pseudo wall formation due to surrounding inflammatory tissue. This was managed conservatively and resolved over a period of time. Figure 7.38 (on DVD): peri-hepatic hypoechoic collection. Figures 7.39 and 7.40 (both on DVD): portal vein thrombosis; US and CT.

Ultrasound thorax

The most common indication for an ultrasound of the thorax is to confirm or estimate the size of pleural effusion. Occasionally ultrasound of the thorax may be required in an ITU setting not only to assess the pleural collection but also guide its drainage [19]. In the accident and emergency department, it is worthwhile scanning the thorax in cases of poly trauma (time permitting!), as chest injuries are often associated with abdominal trauma and hemothorax may be present. Experts also manage to diagnose pneumothorax as rarely a supine CXR may not show the classic features of pneumothorax due to the air rising to the front rather than the apex of the chest.

Technique

The probe most suitable is a 3.5 MHz sector probe, although a curvilinear probe can also be used. Ideally, scanning is carried out with the patient sitting with the probe placed in the intercostal region anteriorly, laterally and posteriorly as show in Figures 7.41 and 7.42 (both on DVD). The scan can be performed at different intercostal levels. However this may be difficult in acutely ill patients in the accident and emergency department and ITU, as the surface area available for scanning may be limited. Under these circumstances, best use of the available area for scanning should be made to gain maximum information. A simple pleural effusion is seen as a homogeneously anechoic area above the liver and diaphragm on the right side and spleen and the diaphragm on the left side. In cases of empyema, pleural fluid may have internal echoes and septations, although simple collections may occasionally

Table 7.8 Checklist for ultrasound of the thorax
• 3.5 MHz sector or curvilinear probe
• Patient sitting if possible
• Anterior, lateral and posterior regions
• Intercostal approach
• Simple fluid seen as anechoic (black)
• Empyema is echogenic and septated
• Underlying lung is collapsed

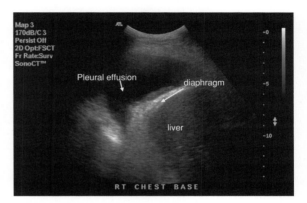

Figures 7.43 Pleural effusion.

be septated. US scan is superior to CT in demonstrating the presence of septations. US scan can also be used to mark the site for drainage or to perform US scan-guided drainage. Loculated effusions can also be better assessed by US scan, but contrast CT may give more information with regard to the location, especially in an immobile patient whose posterior thoracic region cannot be assessed adequately by US scan. An enhancing wall on contrast CT suggests an empyema. Image-guided intervention may be performed using either US or CT to aspirate, drain, insert mini chest tubes, chemical pleurodesis and insert chemotherapeutic agents [19, 20] (Table 7.8).

Figures 7.41 and 7.42 (both on DVD) show the position of the probe for scanning the chest.

Figure 7.43 shows the presence of a right-sided effusion on ultrasound, which is anechoic and there are no septations. Drainage of this led to resolution of the patient's symptoms.

Figures 7.44 and 7.45 (both on DVD): CXR and US showing right-sided effusion. US reveals echogenic contents with septations in a pyrexial patient in keeping with an empyema. A CT was performed.

Figure 7.46 (on DVD) is a CT scan showing the presence of a right-sided collection with locules of air either due to infection or previous attempts at aspiration. The enhancing wall is a feature of empyema. This was drained under CT guidance.

Glossary

(1) Morrison's pouch	the hepato-renal space, which in normal condition does not contain any fluid
(2) Axial	the anatomical cross-section of the human body at right angles to the head to toe plane
(3) Sagittal	the anatomical cross-section at right angles to the right to left (side to side) plane
(4) Coronal	the anatomical cross-section at right angles to the anterior–posterior plane (front to back)
(5) Echogenic	appears bright on USS
(6) Hyperechoic	appears brighter than usual or in comparison to other structures
(7) Hypoechoic	appears less bright or darker than usual or in comparison
(8) Anechoic	no echoes are seen and therefore appear completely dark, e.g. urine in a bladder
(9) Linear probe	straight foot which emits sound waves at right angles. Narrow vertical beam
(10) Curvilinear probe	has a curved (like a sector) foot. Emits sound waves in a diverging sector. Therefore wider view at the depth
(11) Sector probe	has a flat footprint but emits diverging sound waves like a curvilinear probe. Used in areas where space is restricted, such as intercostal space and cranial ultrasound in infants
(12) Doppler	a phenomenon used to assess flow in arteries and veins. But flowing urine can also be seen as jets coming from the reteric orifice in the bladder
(13) 3.5 MHz	is a 3.5 megahertz probe that has greater depth but lesser resolution. Used for all routine abdominal examinations
(14) 5 MHz	5 megahertz probe has higher resolution but less depth. Used for small parts and superficial structures

REFERENCES

1. McGahan JP, Wang L, Richards JR. From the RSNA refresher courses: focused abdominal US for trauma. *Radiographics* 2001;21:S191–9.
2. Habib FA, McKenney MG. Surgeon-performed ultrasound in the ICU setting. *Surgical Clinics of North America* 2004;84(4):1151–79, vii. Review.
3. Rothlin MA, Naf R, Amgwerd M, Candinas D, Frick T, Trentz O. Ultrasound in blunt abdominal and thoracic trauma. *Journal of Trauma* 1993;34:488–95.
4. McGahan JP, Rose J, Coates TL, Wisner DH, Newberry P. Use of ultrasonography in the patient with acute abdominal trauma. *Journal of Ultrasound Medicine* 1997;16:653–62.
5. Sirlin CB, Casola G, Brown MA, Patel N, Bendavid EJ, Hoyt DB. Quantification of fluid on screening ultrasonography for blunt abdominal trauma: a simple scoring system to predict severity of injury. *Journal of Ultrasound Medicine* 2001;20(4):359–64.

6. McGahan Jo, Richards J, Gillen M. The focused abdominal sonography for trauma scan: pearls and pitfalls. *Journal of Ultrasound Medicine* 2002;21:789–800.

7. Miller MT, Pasquale MD, Bromberg WJ, Wasser TE, Cox J. Not so FAST. *Journal of Trauma* 2003;54(1):52–9; discussion 59–60.

8. Pulyert J. Acute appendicitis: US evaluation using graded compression. *Radiology* 1986 Feb;158(2):355–60.

9. Palmer PES. Manual of Diagnostic Ultrasound. Geneva, WHO. 1995;55.

10. McGregor JC, Pollock JG, Anton HC. The diagnosis and assessment of abdominal aortic aneurysms by ultrasonography. *Annals of the Royal College of Surgeons of England* 1976;58(5):388–92.

11. Bennett GL, Balthazar EJ. Ultrasound and CT evaluation of emergent gallbladder pathology. *Radiology Clinics of North America* 2003;41(6):1203–16. Review.

12. Hanbidge AE, Buckler PM, O'Malley ME, Wilson SR. From the RSNA refresher courses: imaging evaluation for acute pain in the right upper quadrant. *Radiographics* 2004; 24(4):1117–35.

13. Boland GW, Slater G, Lu DS, Eisenberg P, Lee MJ, Mueller PR. Prevalence and significance of gallbladder abnormalities seen on sonography in intensive care unit patients. *American Journal of Roentgenology* 2000; 174(4):973–7.

14. Wong CH, Trinh TM, Robbins AN, Rowen SJ, Cohen AJ. Diagnosis of appendicitis: imaging findings in patients with atypical clinical features. *American Journal of Roentgenology* 1993;161(6):1199–203.

15. Parulekar SG. Ultrasonographic findings in diseases of the appendix. *Journal of Ultrasound Medicine* 1983;2(2):59–64.

16. Ajayi AT, Adejuyigbe O, Makanjuola D. Radiologic and sonographic evaluation of intra-abdominal abscesses in a Nigerian population. *East African Medical Journal* 1993;70(9):540–3.

17. Golding RH, Li DK, Cooperberg PL. Sonographic demonstration of air–fluid levels in abdominal abscesses. *Journal of Ultrasound Medicine* 1982;1(4):151–5.

18. Men S, Akhan O, Koroglu M. Percutaneous drainage of abdominal abscess. *European Journal of Radiology* 2002;43(3):204–18.

19. Beagle GL. Bedside diagnostic ultrasound and therapeutic ultrasound-guided procedures in the intensive care setting. *Critical Care Clinics* 2000;16(1):59–81.

20. Moulton JS. Image-guided management of complicated pleural fluid collections. *Radiology Clinics of North America* 2000;38(2): 345–74.

ACKNOWLEDGMENT

The authors are grateful to Tony Bailey for the line illustrations.

Chapter 8

Use of ultrasound to aid local anesthetic nerve blocks in adults

BARRY NICHOLLS, STEPHAN KAPRAL, PETER MARHOFER AND ALICE ROBERTS

Part 1

Introduction

Regional anesthesia involves the placement of local anesthetic close to a nerve or plexus to block transmission of the nerve(s), thereby achieving anesthesia of the area of innervation of the nerve/plexus. The area of anesthesia is dependent on the nerve(s) blocked, being as little as a finger (digital nerve block), the whole arm (brachial plexus block) or the lower half of the body (spinal/epidural). The advantages of these techniques are the anesthesia or analgesia that they achieve (loss of sensation or absence of pain in the area of operation or injury). These techniques can be employed on their own for limited surgery (brachial plexus for arm surgery, epidural or spinal for hip surgery), or in combination with general anesthesia for more extensive surgery. Depending on the local anesthetic used (Lidocaine, short acting; Bupivacaine, long acting), the anesthesia and analgesia can be extended into the post-operative period for 4–12 h, and if catheters are left in place (a thin plastic catheter <20 g within a plexus or beside a nerve) for up to 3–4 days.

Identification of the nerve

The success of any of these techniques relies on the accurate location and identification of the nerve or plexus. Early attempts at regional anesthesia (Halsted in 1884) employed surgical exposure of the brachial plexus and direct injection of local anesthetic (cocaine) into the nerve roots. The success and complications of these techniques are unknown, but this approach rapidly lost favor with the introduction of the hypodermic needle and the development of percutaneous techniques based on anatomy and superficial landmarks. Almost all the present-day techniques were developed in the early part of the twentieth century: supraclavicular approach (Kulenkampff, 1911); axillary approach (Hirschel, 1911); and infraclavicular (Bazy, 1914). Although minor modifications have taken place over the subsequent years, e.g. axillary (Reding, 1921; Eriksson, 1962), the common approaches have changed little since their inception. This is a testament to the fact that the anatomy of the human body has not changed since regional anesthesia started, only the ability to image and localize each nerve has improved.

Initially, localization of the nerve/plexus was achieved by either paresthesia (direct contact of the nerve with the needle) or specific endpoint identification (loss of resistance, bony contact). With the improved development of needle technology and the increased interest in the use of electrical nerve stimulation techniques following Melzack

Ultrasound in Anesthetic Practice, ed. Graham Arthurs and Barry Nicholls. Published by Cambridge University Press.
© Cambridge University Press 2009.

and Wall gate theory published in 1965, peripheral nerve stimulation for regional anesthesia developed. Peripheral nerve stimulation (PNS) has been the primary method of nerve location and identification for the past 30 years, relying on the inverse relationship of current and distance to the nerve to place a needle close to the target nerve.

Peripheral nerve stimulation

Peripheral nerve simulation (PNS) will reliably identify a nerve by causing depolarization of the nerve. This causes contraction in the muscles supplied by the nerve, e.g. biceps stimulated by the musculocutaneous nerve. It is important when using PNS not only to know what muscles are supplied by which nerves, but also the response of these muscles, e.g. elbow flexion–biceps–musculocutaneous nerve. Most nerves are mixed nerves (sensory and motor) and identification of the motor response will be followed by a combined sensory and motor blockade after injection of local anesthetic. The success of PNS is dependent on how close the needle can be positioned next to the nerve. The current needed to stimulate the nerve is inversely proportional to the distance of the needle to the nerve. This means that the closer the needle is to the nerve, the less current is needed to stimulate it. It is generally accepted that a current of between 0.3 and 0.5 mA is ideal, correlating to the needle being approximately 1–2 mm from the nerve. Currents of less than 0.2 mA are to be avoided, as they could indicate that the needle is touching or within the nerve and as such may increase the likelihood of nerve damage.

All techniques so far described have one thing in common: they are "blind" techniques, relying on mechanisms of paresthesia and motor responses to position the needle as close to the target nerve/plexus as possible. They both assume that the local anesthetic once injected will always spread uniformly around the nerve and that the nerves will always be exactly where they are meant to be. As a result of these misconceptions, regional anesthesia at present has a built in failure rate of 5–20%. This failure rate can be reduced by close attention to detail and experience, but not completely eliminated.

It is important to realize that the needle does not block the nerve but the local anesthetic, and unless you can either accurately predict the spread or visualize the spread, there will always be a failure rate in the above blind techniques. Also anatomical variation is extremely common; the roots, cord and divisions of the brachial plexus may join, divide and separate at different levels.

Imaging techniques

Imaging techniques can improve our understanding of anatomy and anatomical variance, confirm proposed needle trajectories and examine the extent of local anesthetic spread (dye studies). However, their use in clinical anesthesia is limited both by radiation exposure (X-ray, CT) and their immovable size and magnetism (CT and MRI).

Ultrasound

Ultrasound uses 2D imaging techniques for the real-time visualization of structures and has the potential to revolutionize regional anesthesia.

In the 1980s, a Doppler ultrasound probe was used initially to help locate subclavian and axillary vessels to assist with supraclavicular and axillary techniques. Since the 1990s, it has developed into a specific stand-alone technique. The development of smaller, more powerful portable machines has seen the widespread proliferation of this technique in normal clinical practice, with ultrasound now seen as the natural successor to peripheral nerve stimulation. Ultrasound appears to fulfill all the criteria for predictable regional anesthetic success, e.g. real-time visualization of the nerve, direct observation and guidance of the needle to the nerve, and confirmation of the spread of local anesthetic.

Preliminary studies have confirmed improved success rates, reduced volumes of local anesthetic needed, faster performance times, decreased latency of onset, reduced paresthesia and vascular puncture and improved patient comfort.

General principles of ultrasound applicable to regional anesthesia

Ultrasound is a highly operator-dependent imaging modality; it is not enough just to have an understanding of physics and the machine's capabilities. To recognize the structures and interpret the image, a detailed knowledge of anatomy is essential. It is also important to understand how to obtain and capture an image, differentiate true image from artifact, and understand how the interaction between the tissues and ultrasound may affect the picture (i.e. not all patients give good images). Even after this has been understood, the operator needs to be able to maintain a stable image and introduce a needle; placing it close to the nerve/plexus and avoiding other important structures (arteries, veins and lung).

There are three important components required, for this to be achieved.

(1) Image capture.
(2) Image interpretation.
(3) Needling techniques.

Image capture

The optimization of the image depends on a number of factors including the machine used, choice of probe, acoustic coupling of probe to skin, hand movements, and adjustment of image with respect to gain, focus and depth. Knowledge is needed of the physical interaction of the sound beam and the tissues and how it may affect the picture, e.g. reflection, attenuation, artifacts and the anisotropic properties of the structures being visualized.

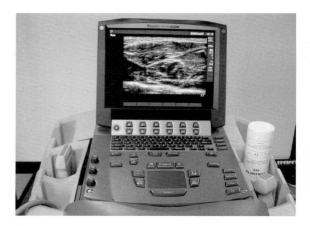

Figure 8.1.1　Sonosite MicroMaxx.

Machine

Cart-based radiology and cardiology machines are expensive and rarely seen outside of radiology and cardiology departments. As such, they initially restricted both the enthusiasm and accessibility of ultrasound into anesthesia. Over the past five years, smaller portable machines have become available. These machines initially had limited functions and gave poor picture quality, but now there are a number of good quality, portable "laptop" machines available (Sonosite®: Micromaxx (Figure 8.1.1), Esaote® Mylabs and GE® LogicE). These machines have Doppler, tissue harmonics and multi-beam technology as standard, making them a true alternative to the traditional cart-based machine.

Probe

Depending on the area being imaged and the depth of the structures, a variety of probes may be used (Figure 8.1.2). As a general rule, use the highest frequency probe available for the depth of the target you want to image. With this in mind, resolution is best at higher frequencies, but the higher frequencies are attenuated more as they pass through the tissues, limiting the depth of vision. High-frequency probes are best for superficial or small structures (brachial plexus, peripheral nerves) and

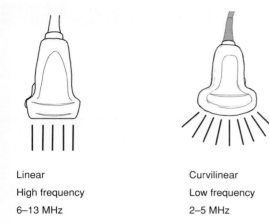

Linear
High frequency
6–13 MHz

Curvilinear
Low frequency
2–5 MHz

Figure 8.1.2   Linear and curvilinear probes.

low-frequency probes for deep or large structures (sciatic nerve, lumbar plexus). The probe's "footprint" (size of the probe face) may limit access and view (supraclavicular, pediatric cases), and in these cases smaller probes may be necessary.

Acoustic coupling

Ultrasound cannot pass through air. It is imperative that there is no air between the probe face and the skin. To achieve this, an acoustic coupling is used; commonly, this is ultrasound (water-based) gel. A disposable probe cover is used to protect the probe from contamination and to maintain sterility when used for performing practical procedures.

Hand movements

Once the probe is lightly applied to the skin, three basic hand movements are employed to improve view and find the target (Figure 8.1.3).

(a) Slide. A movement up and down the skin (distal/proximal), following structure(s) identifying branching or optimal entry point.

(b) Tilting. A rocking hand movement, to optimize angle of insonation and to obtain the best view of the structure. This is also useful when the nerve is varying its depth.

(c) Rotating. A twisting movement, to obtain the true short axis view of the nerve and vessels: when an artery or vein is round not oval.

Image adjustment

All machines are different, and it is important to understand which knob does what (knobology) before using them. All machines will allow adjustment of depth (Figure 8.1.4, on DVD) and gain (Figure 8.1.5, on DVD); changing the focus may be optional, allowing a number of areas of focus to be achieved or as with Sonosite machines fixed: focus is set to the middle of the screen.

Depth should be adjusted so that the target structure is in the middle of the screen, with gain being adjusted so that contrast is consistent throughout the screen. Echoes of similar structures give rise to similar screen brightness regardless of their depth.

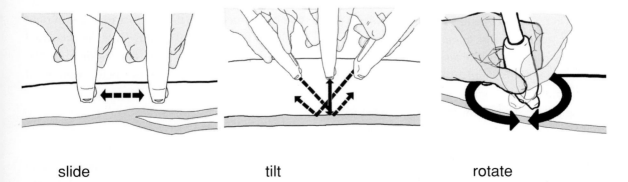

slide   tilt   rotate

Figure 8.1.3   Hand movements.

Table 8.1.1 Sonographic appearances of peripheral nerves and surrounding tissues

Tissue	Ultrasound appearance
ARTERIES	Anechoic (black circles – tubes) – pulsatile
VEINS	Anechoic (black circles – tubes) – compressible
TENDONS Fibrillar appearance	**Longitudinal** – tubular structure Internal architecture, loosely packed continuous blurred bright lines (hyperechoic), pale surface **Transverse** circular structure with pale halo (tendon sheath) Internal architecture hyperechoic (semi-bright) dots (tendon fibrils) loosely packed, within hypoechoic (darkened) surroundings – granular appearance Anisotropic ++
NERVES Fascicular appearance	**Longitudinal** – tubular structures– bright surface Internal architecture multiple broken bright (hyperechoic) lines **Transverse** – circular structure with bright surface (epineurium) Internal architecture multiple hypoechoic black dots (nerve fascicles) with bright outlines within bright surroundings (connective tissue, perineurium) Speckled appearance Anisotropic +
PLEURA	Hyperechoic line(s) – sliding lung sign with respiration
LUNG	Not visualized due to air/gray lines – reverberation artifacts from pleura
BONES Periosteum cortex and medulla	Hyperechoic ++ line Anechoic – black (drop-down shadowing – due to reflection of beam by periosteum)

Tissue interaction and artifacts

Ultrasound waves are similar to all longitudinal waves including light; they undergo reflection, scattering, refraction and attenuation, all of which may influence the image obtained. Specular reflection (mirror reflection) forms the basis of the ultrasound image and will occur at all tissue interfaces; scatter and refraction depend very much on the tissues encountered; and attenuation is very much frequency-dependent. The resultant image is a mixture of true reflection and artifact; it is important to understand and recognize common artifacts, including post-cystic enhancement (Figure 8.1.6, on DVD), lateral shadowing, and needle reverberation.

Anisotropy

This is the single most important artifact or concept of physics that needs to be understood when imaging nerves. For certain tissues, e.g. nerves and tendons, the angle of insonation (angle of the ultrasound beam to the structure) will have a tremendous influence on the reflection and the consequent image obtained. This is a complex relationship between the frequency of the beam and the tissues being imaged. For nerves, the best picture is obtained when the nerves are imaged at right angles to the beam (90°) as the angle is decreased the visibility decreases and changes of only 10–20° may result in the nerve not being seen at all (Figure 8.1.7).

Image interpretation

Ultrasound images are black and white, and differentiating between different types of tissues (Table 8.1.1), e.g. muscle, fat and vessels, involves not only pattern recognition but also observing their

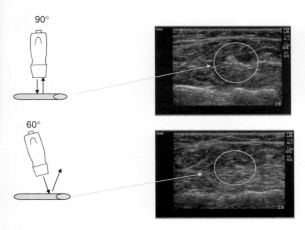

Figure 8.1.7   Anisotropy.

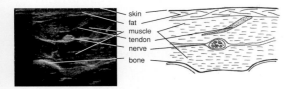

Figure 8.1.8   Ultrasound appearance of tissues.

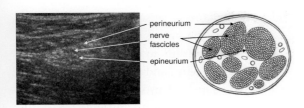

Figure 8.1.9   Short axis scan of peripheral nerve.

real-time interaction with the ultrasound probe and beam (compression, pulsation, anisotropy and Doppler shift) (Figure 8.1.8).

Each peripheral nerve is a collection of motor and sensory axons arranged into fascicles within connective tissue accompanied by arteries and veins all enclosed within a protective sheath. As such they have distinctive ultrasound appearances – "speckled" or "fascicular" (Figures 8.1.9 and 8.1.10).

The appearance of peripheral nerves does, however, vary considerably, being round, ovoid tri-

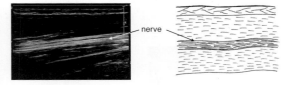

Figure 8.1.10   Long axis scan of peripheral nerve.

angular and occasionally flattened depending on their surrounding structures (compression). Their echogenicity also varies, being relatively hypo-echoic (interscalene – black holes/bubbles) or hyperechoic (sciatic – bright structure). This may be influenced by:

- size of the nerve;
- structural appearance (histological): some nerves have a lot of connective tissue, e.g. epineurium, perineurium;
- depth from the skin;
- probe design (linear or curvilinear). Frequency of beam (MHz);
- Angle of incidence of beam: certain nerves are highly anisotropic, e.g. sciatic nerve;
- surrounding structures (large muscles attenuate the ultrasound beam, leading to reduced visibility, e.g. sciatic nerve.

Needling techniques

It is important when performing practical procedures that the needle tip is visualized at all times. All needles show up equally well with ultrasound, albeit larger needles give a brighter reflection and certain tip designs may help (Tuohy) – initially use a needle you are comfortable with. Short beveled needles are preferable to long beveled needles, as they have a better "feel", and the injection port is at the tip of the needle, making it more difficult to position intraneurally in a longer needle.

The needle can be introduced either in:

- Out-of-plane (OOP) approach: at right angles to the long axis of the probe (across the probe); the

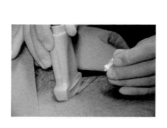
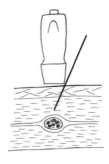

Figure 8.1.11 Out-of-plane approach of needle.

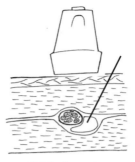
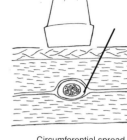

Unilateral spread
(reposition needle)

Circumferential spread
(donut sign)

Figure 8.1.13 Spread of local anesthetic solution.

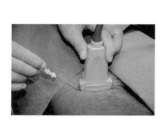
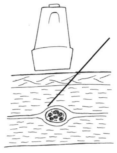

Figure 8.1.12 In-plane approach of needle.

needle will only be visible when it crosses the beam.

CAUTION: always identify the tip of the needle and follow with the US (Figure 8.1.11).

- In-plane (IP) approach: along the long axis of the probe (parallel to the probe face); the needle will be visualized throughout its entire length (Figure 8.1.12).

Needle to nerve position

It is important not to deliberately contact the nerve, both to reduce the likelihood of damage, but also for patient comfort. Position the needle close to the nerve (the identity of the nerve can be confirmed using peripheral nerve stimulation), and then inject a small volume of local anesthetic, observing its spread. Spread of local anesthetic should ideally encircle the nerve (Figure 8.1.13 needle nerve position).

Practical application of ultrasound in regional anesthesia

- Place probe lightly on skin over the target plexus or nerve, ensuring an air-free contact using gel or alcohol spray.
- Orientate probe, so as to mirror hand movements (all probes have a mark which corresponds to a dot on the screen).
- Identify a landmark: vessel or muscle.
- Gently move the probe, visualizing the target, noting its relationship to other important structures (arteries, veins, and pleura).
- Gentle pressure will usually distinguish arteries from veins (arteries: pulsatile anechoic; veins: compressible anechoic). Color Doppler or power Doppler will distinguish vessels from nerves.
- With the target in the middle of the screen, gentle pressure on the skin will help to determine the optimum entry point. Infiltrate the skin with local anesthetic.
- Clean site with alcohol solution (70% isopropyl alcohol), drape, and cover probe with sterile probe cover. Apply sterile ultrasound gel (or use alcohol solution) to achieve an air-free contact between probe and skin.
- Air is the worst medium for ultrasound (99% of the beam is reflected from an air–tissue interface,

obscuring any view of deeper structures). It is important to ensure an adequate layer of gel on the probe and remove all air from the injectate (whiteout).

- Using a needle of your choice (insulated or uninsulated), introduce the needle in either the in-plane or out-of-plane approach.
- After passing through the skin, identify the needle within the US beam; always find the needle with the probe, NEVER the probe with the needle.
- Direct the needle towards the target, position the needle beside the nerve (do not deliberately contact the nerve).
- A peripheral nerve stimulator can be used in conjunction with the US. This confirms the position and identity of the nerve and aids in teaching.
- Inject local anesthetic (2 ml aliquots). Observe spread of solution (encircling nerve) and, if unacceptable, reposition needle under direct vision and re-inject.

Golden rules

(1) Never advance the needle unless you can identify the needle tip.
(2) Never deliberately contact the nerve: place the needle next to the nerve.
(3) Observe injection: if unable to see spread of local anesthetic, consider intravascular injection/needle not in scan plane.
(4) If the nerve swells on injection, stop and consider intraneural injection.
(5) Injection should be resistance-free and painless; if not, STOP and reposition needle.

FURTHER READING

1. Marhofer P, Greher M, Kapral S. Ultrasound guidance in regional anaesthesia. *British Journal of Anaesthesia* 2005 Jan; 94(1):7–17.
2. Retz G, Kapral S, Greher M, Mauritz W. Ultrasound findings of the axillary part of the brachial plexus. *Anesthesia and Analgesia* 2001;92:1271–5.
3. Scafhalter-Zoppoth I, McCulloch C, Gray AT. Ultrasound visibility of needles used for regional nerve block: an in vitro study. *Regional Anesthesia and Pain Medicine* 2004 Sep–Oct;29(5):480–8.
4. Williams SR, Chouinard P, Arcand G, *et al.* Ultrasound guidance speeds execution and improves quality of supraclavicular block. *Anesthesia and Analgesia* 2003 Nov;97(5): 1518–23.
5. Perlas A, Chan VW, Simons M. Brachial plexus examination and electrical stimulation: a volunteer study. *Anesthesiology* 2003 Aug;(2):429–35.
6. Sandhu NS, Capan LM. Ultrasound-guided infraclavicular brachial plexus block. *British Journal of Anaesthesia* 2002 Aug;89:254–9.

Part 2: Anatomical background to upper limb blockade

Brachial plexus
Anatomy of the brachial plexus
The roots of the brachial plexus from the anterior primary rami of spinal nerves C5–T1 emerge from the cervical intervertebral foramina to lie between the anterior and middle scalene muscles.

The phrenic nerve (C3,4,5: derived from the roots of both cervical and brachial plexi) winds forwards and medially from the interscalene groove, across the anterior scalene muscle to disappear into the thorax and supply the diaphragm. Two nerves branch from the roots: the dorsal scapular nerve (C5) pierces the middle scalene muscle, then runs deep to levator scapulae to innervate the rhomboid muscles attaching to the medial border of the scapula; the long thoracic nerve (C5,6, and C7 in 40%) also runs posteriorly to the plexus and pierces the middle scalene muscle, descending onto the

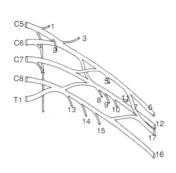

1. Dorsal scapular nerve
2. Nerve to subclavius
3. Suprascapular nerve
4. Long thoracic nerve
5. Lateral pectoral nerve
6. Musculocutaneous nerve
7. Lateral root – median nerve

8. Upper subscapular nerve
9. Thoracodorsal nerve
10. Lower subscapular nerve
11. Axillary nerve
12. Radial nerve

13. Medial pectoral nerve
14. Medial cut nerve of arm
15. Medial cut nerve of forearm
16. Ulnar
17. Medial root – median nerve

Figure 8.2.1   Brachial plexus line drawing.

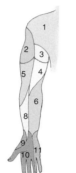
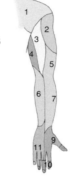

1. Lateral supraclavicular nerves .1
2. Axillary .2
3. Intercosto-brachial .3
4. Medial cut nerve of arm .4
5. Lateral cutaneous nerve of arm .5
6. Medial cut nerve of forearm .6
7. Posterior cut nerve of forearm .7
8. Lateral cut nerve of forearm .8
9. Radial .9
10. Median .10
11. Ulnar .11

Figure 8.2.2   Cutaneous nerves of the arm.

chest wall (the medial wall of the axilla) to supply serratus anterior muscle. The nerve to subclavius (C5,6) is referred to as either a low branch from the roots or a high branch from the upper trunk; it descends anterior to the plexus to innervate subclavius muscle under the clavicle (Figures 8.2.1 and 8.2.2.).

Interscalene
The anatomy of the groove
The interscalene groove lies between the anterior and middle scalene muscles, which attach from the cervical vertebrae to the first rib. These muscles are therefore anterior and lateral flexors of the neck, as well as being accessory muscles of respiration (as they may act to lift the first rib if the

neck is fixed in position). The subclavian artery lies in the lowest part of the interscalene groove, and the brachial plexus lies lateral and posterior to the artery. The interscalene groove can be palpated in the neck, with the fingers resting on the posterior border of sternocleidomastoid muscle, just superior to the clavicle, and then allowed to drop posteriorly onto the floor of the posterior triangle of the neck. The interscalene groove is then felt about 1 cm behind the posterior border of sternocleidomastoid. It is easiest to feel if the patient lies supine and is then asked to lift their head from the pillow, thus contracting and accentuating the sternocleidomastoid. In the most inferior part of the interscalene groove, the pulsation of the subclavian artery will be felt as it is pushed against the first rib. The brachial plexus itself may be felt just posterior and lateral to the artery. As it is palpated, the patient will usually feel a slightly unpleasant twinge (Figure 8.2.3).

The interscalene groove represents the point at which the brachial plexus emerges into the floor of the posterior triangle of the neck. As the roots emerge from the interscalene groove, they combine to form the trunks of the brachial plexus: C5 and C6 root join to form the upper trunk; C7 root continues as the middle trunk; C8 and T1 join to form the lower trunk. These trunks lie on the levator scapulae muscle, and deep to the prevertebral fascia of the neck; it is this fascia which will be projected to form a sheath around them – and the subclavian artery – as the brachial plexus runs into the axilla. The trunks are crossed superficially by the supraclavicular nerves, the nerve to subclavius, the inferior belly of omohyoid, the external jugular vein, and the superficial branch of the transverse cervical artery.

Supraclavicular
The anatomy of the area
Here, the trunks of the brachial plexus are running across the floor of the base of the posterior

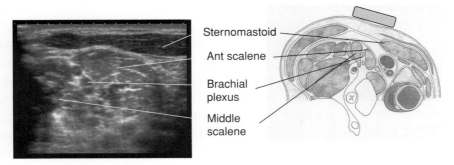

Figure 8.2.3   Interscalene block.

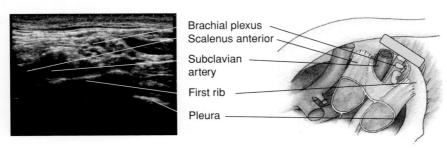

Figure 8.2.4   Supraclavicular block.

triangle, just superior to the clavicle, and eventually disappearing under it as the plexus heads for the axilla and upper limb. A single nerve takes its origin from the upper trunk: the suprascapular nerve (C5, C6) (the only sensory nerve to emerge form above the clavicle), supplying the supraspinatus and infraspinatus muscles, the shoulder and acromioclavicular joints. There are no branches from the middle or lower trunk.

The trunks course down over the first rib, posterior and lateral to the subclavian artery, with the artery separated from the vein anteriorly by the insertion of scalenus anterior. As the three trunks pass deep to the clavicle, they each divide into an anterior and a posterior division; there are no direct branches from the divisions (Figure 8.2.4).

apex of the axillary pyramid), the divisions of the brachial plexus unite to form the cords. The order of the main neurovascular structures passing from the neck into the apex of the axilla is as follows: the subclavian vein (which runs behind the anterior scalene in the neck) is the most anteromedial structure; the subclavian artery lies posterior to the vein; the cords of the brachial plexus lie posterior and lateral to the artery (in the same fascial sheath as the artery). The cords are formed from the divisions as follows: the anterior divisions of the upper and middle trunk unite to form the lateral cord; the anterior division of the lower trunk continues alone as the medial cord; all three posterior divisions unite to form the posterior cord (Figures 8.2.5 and 8.2.6, both on DVD).

Infraclavicular
The anatomy of the area

Just below the lateral part of the clavicle and at the lateral border of the first rib (i.e. in the

Axillary
The anatomy of the mid area

The pectoralis minor muscle is used as the anatomical landmark, dividing the axillary artery into three parts: the first part above the upper border of the pectoralis minor, the second part behind the muscle, and the third part below its inferior border. The lateral and posterior cords of the brachial plexus both lie lateral to the first part of the axillary artery, whilst the medial cord lies posterior. By the second part of the axillary artery, the cords of the brachial plexus have become arranged around the artery according to their names. Thus the medial cord comes to lie medial to the artery, the lateral cord lateral to it, and the large posterior cord behind it, still all enclosed within the same fascial sheath (Figure 8.2.6, on DVD).

The earliest branches to emerge from the cords of the brachial plexus are those supplying the muscles of the shoulder and the walls of the axilla, as well as two cutaneous nerves of the upper limb. Pectoralis major and minor form the anterior wall of the axilla, and are supplied by high branches from the lateral and medial cords: the lateral pectoral nerve (C5,6,7) and medial pectoral nerve (C8, T1), respectively. Two cutaneous nerves – the medial cutaneous nerves of the arm and forearm (both C8, T1) – emerge from the medial cord below the medial pectoral nerve, and descend into the arm medially, leaving the axillary sheath to become more superficial. The medial cutaneous nerve of the arm communicates with the intercostobrachial nerve (from T2) and supplies the distal medial third of the arm, just above the elbow. The medial cutaneous nerve of the forearm supplies the skin over biceps in the arm, and proceeds to supply the skin of the antero-medial forearm, as far as the wrist.

The posterior wall of the axilla is formed by subscapularis muscle, on the deep surface of the scapula, and this is supplied by upper and lower subscapular nerves (C5,6) from the posterior cord. Between these nerves, the thoracodorsal nerve (C6,7,8) emerges from the posterior cord, to supply the latissimus dorsi. The tendon of this muscle forms the posterior wall of the axilla and runs laterally to insert in the intertubercular sulcus of the humerus.

The posterior cord effectively terminates by dividing into the axillary nerve (C5,6) and the larger radial nerve (C5–T1). The axillary nerve disappears posteriorly out of the axilla through the quadrangular space between the tendons of teres minor and major, with the posterior circumflex humeral vessels. This nerve supplies the teres minor and deltoid muscles, the shoulder joint, and also supplies skin over the shoulder, as the upper lateral cutaneous nerve of the arm. The radial nerve leaves the axilla later, through the triangular space, between the tendons of teres major and the short head of triceps brachii, to lie between the medial and lateral heads of triceps, in the radial (or spiral) groove on the posterior surface of the humerus. As it passes through the triangular space, the radial nerve gives branches to the triceps and also gives rise to the posterior cutaneous nerve of the arm.

The lateral cord terminates by dividing into the musculocutaneous nerve and the lateral root of the median nerve (both carrying fibers from C5,6 and 7). The musculocutaneous nerve pierces coracobrachialis muscle, supplying it, then emerges to lie deep to biceps brachii muscle, on brachialis, also supplying both these muscles. It eventually emerges lateral to the tendon of biceps brachii above the elbow, having distributed all of its motor fibers to become the purely sensory lateral cutaneous nerve of the forearm.

The medial cord ends by dividing into the ulnar nerve, which runs medially down the arm, and the medial root of the median nerve, which crosses anterior to the axillary artery to join the lateral root. The root value of the ulnar nerve is usually C7, 8, T1, as it receives some C7 fibers from the lateral root of the median nerve (Figure 8.2.7).

The anatomy of the midhumeral area

Around the midhumeral level, the radial nerve is lying in the spiral or radial groove on the

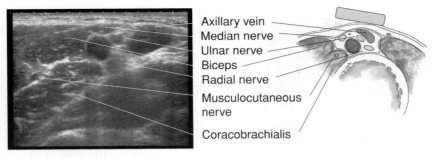

Figure 8.2.7 Axillary approach to brachial plexus.

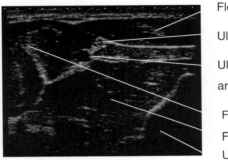

Figure 8.2.9 Ulnar nerve.

posterior surface of the humerus. The radial nerve runs inferolaterally in this groove and eventually pierces the lateral intermuscular septum to enter the anterior compartment of the arm (and will therefore lie anterior to the elbow). The ulnar nerve, having started in the anterior compartment, leaves it by piercing the medial intermuscular septum (to lie posteriorly at the elbow, behind the medial epicondyle). The median nerve, having been formed on the lateral side of the axillary artery, crosses the artery at the midhumeral level, to lie medial to the brachial artery in the cubital fossa. The medial cutaneous nerves of the arm and forearm lie superficially on the medial side of the arm at this level. The musculocutaneous nerve lies deep in the anterior compartment, sandwiched between biceps brachii and brachialis muscles. The musculocutaneous nerve gives off a branch, the lateral cutaneous nerve of the forearm, which emerges lateral to the tendon of biceps, becoming superficial, and runs down into the forearm (Figure 8.2.8, on DVD).

The anatomy of the elbow and forearm

At the elbow, the ulnar nerve lies posterior to the medial epicondyle. The median nerve lies in the cubital fossa, medial to the brachial artery, and at this point gives branches to four of the five superficial forearm flexor muscles (pronator teres, flexor carpi radialis, palmaris longus, and flexor digitorum superficialis). The radial nerve lies lateral to the tendon of biceps brachii, and here divides into its terminal branches: the superficial radial nerve and the posterior interosseous nerve.

Ulnar nerve

The ulnar nerve passes between the heads of flexor carpi ulnaris (fcu) into the anterior compartment of the forearm, running down between fcu and the deep flexor digitorum profundus (fdp). It supplies fcu (the fifth superficial forearm muscle) and, in most cases, the medial two muscle bellies of fdp (Figure 8.2.9).

101

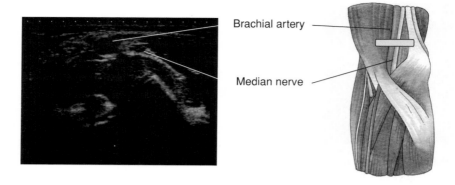

Figure 8.2.10   Median nerve.

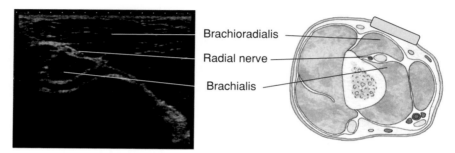

Figure 8.2.11   Radial nerve.

Median nerve

The median nerve gives its branches to the superficial forearm flexors, then runs deep, disappearing out of the cubital fossa by passing between the two heads of pronator teres, then running under the fibrous arch of flexor digitorum superficialis. It gives a deeper branch, the anterior interosseous nerve, which lies on the surface of the interosseous membrane, deep to the deep flexors (Figure 8.2.10).

Radial nerve

The superficial radial nerve remains in the anterior compartment of the forearm, running just beneath the border of brachioradialis, then under the brachioradialis tendon near the wrist, and into the anatomical snuffbox, where it becomes superficial. The posterior interosseous nerve is destined to supply the forearm extensors; it passes posteriorly, between the heads of supinator, to lie on the posterior aspect of the interosseous membrane and supply the posterior compartment (Figure 8.2.11).

The anatomy of the wrist and hand
Ulnar nerve

At the wrist, the ulnar nerve lies just radial to the tendon of fcu, between this tendon and the ulnar artery. The artery and nerve pass into the hand superficial to the flexor retinaculum; the ulnar nerve is therefore spared in carpal tunnel syndrome. The ulnar nerve gives palmar cutaneous branches to the hypothenar skin, superficial branches to palmaris brevis and the medial one and a half fingers (digital nerves), and deep branches to the intrinsic muscles of the hand.

Median nerve

The median nerve lies almost centrally at the wrist, between the tendons of flexor carpi radialis and flexor digitorum superficialis, beneath and slightly radial to the more superficial tendon of palmaris longus. Just proximal to the wrist, the median nerve gives off a superficial palmar branch, which supplies skin over the base of the palm and thenar eminence. The median nerve itself then passes under the flexor retinaculum, through the tightly packed carpal tunnel, into the hand. Once into the hand, recurrent branches of the median nerve supply the muscles of the thenar eminence, and the remaining nerve divides into a medial and lateral branch, forming common digital nerves (to the radial three and a half digits) running between the digits. These divide near the web spaces into proper digital nerves, running along the sides of each finger (Figure 8.2.12, on DVD).

Radial nerve

The radial nerve runs deep to the tendon of brachioradialis near the wrist, running dorsally into the anatomical snuffbox (the triangular depression between the tendons of abductor pollucis longus, extensor pollucis brevis and extensor pollucis longus). It breaks into terminal branches, which spread out superficially over the tendon of extensor pollucis longus (where they may be palpated) and supply the skin of the radial side of the dorsum of the hand.

Part 3: Anatomical background to lower limb blockade

Lumbar plexus
The anatomy and sonoanatomy of the lumbosacral plexus

The lumbar plexus represents the upper part of the plexus supplying the lower limb, the lower part being the sacral plexus within the pelvis. The lumbar plexus is formed from the anterior primary rami of lumbar spinal nerves 1–4, which emerge from the intervertebral foramina of the lumbar spine to lie within the psoas major muscle, between the anterior and posterior masses of the muscle. These anterior primary rami give segmental branches to the psoas and quadratus lumborum, then form the lumbar plexus (Figures 8.3.1 and 8.3.2).

Ilioinguinal and iliohypogastric nerves

The first branch of the lumbar plexus is part of the L1 anterior primary ramus, which supplies the anterolateral abdominal wall, as the lowest of a series of nerves, which begin with the anterior primary ramus of T7, supplying the epigastric region. The L1 anterior primary ramus divides to create the iliohypogastric nerve and its collateral,

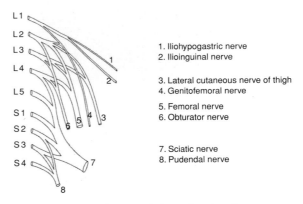

1. Iliohypogastric nerve
2. Ilioinguinal nerve

3. Lateral cutaneous nerve of thigh
4. Genitofemoral nerve

5. Femoral nerve
6. Obturator nerve

7. Sciatic nerve
8. Pudendal nerve

Figure 8.3.1 Lumbar-sacral plexus line drawing.

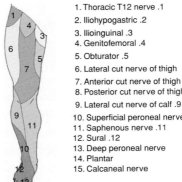
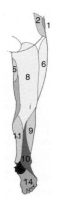

1. Thoracic T12 nerve .1
2. Iliohypogastric .2
3. Ilioinguinal .3
4. Genitofemoral .4
5. Obturator .5
6. Lateral cut nerve of thigh
7. Anterior cut nerve of thigh .7
8. Posterior cut nerve of thigh .8
9. Lateral cut nerve of calf .9
10. Superficial peroneal nerve .10
11. Saphenous nerve .11
12. Sural .12
13. Deep peroneal nerve
14. Plantar
15. Calcaneal nerve

Figure 8.3.2 Cutaneous nerves of the leg.

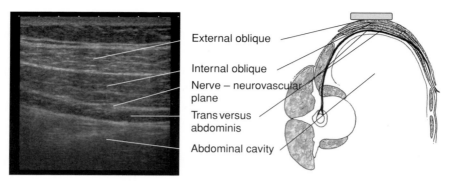

Figure 8.3.3 Abdominal wall.

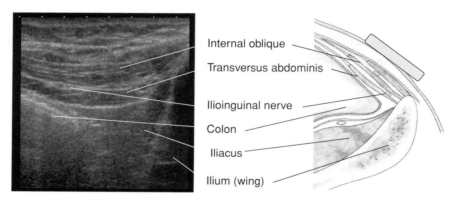

Figure 8.3.4 Ilioinguinal nerve.

the ilioinguinal nerve. The iliohypogastric nerve emerges from the psoas, just beneath the subcostal nerve (the T12 anterior primary ramus) and runs across the quadratus lumborum, retroperitoneally. It runs laterally through the transversus abdominis muscle and into the neurovascular plane between this muscle and the internal oblique. A lateral cutaneous branch pierces the oblique abdominal muscles to supply the skin of the upper buttock. The iliohypogastric nerve continues running anteriorly. It pierces the internal oblique above and about 2 cm medial to the anterior superior iliac spine, and the external oblique about 3 cm above the superficial inguinal ring (5 cm above the pubic tubercle), to supply the skin of the suprapubic area (Figure 8.3.3).

The ilioinguinal nerve initially runs just below the iliohypogastric nerve, in the neurovascular plane between the transversus abdominis and the internal oblique muscles, giving branches to the lower fibers of these muscles. It then pierces the internal oblique to enter the inguinal canal, where it runs underneath the spermatic cord to the superficial inguinal ring. It supplies a small area of skin on the upper thigh, just below the pubic tubercle. The ilioinguinal nerve descends with the spermatic cord, within the external spermatic fascia, piercing this fascial layer to supply the skin over the root of the penis and the anterior third of the scrotum in the male, or the mons pubis and anterior third of the labia majora in the female (Figure 8.3.4).

Lower limb
Genitofemoral nerve

The genitofemoral nerve (L1,2) runs through the substance of the psoas to emerge on its anterior

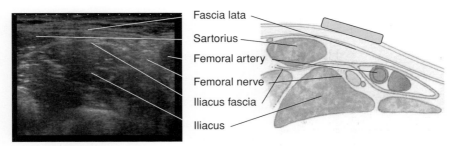

Fascia lata
Sartorius
Femoral artery
Femoral nerve
Iliacus fascia
Iliacus

Figure 8.3.5   Femoral nerve.

surface. It then runs down on this muscle, dividing into genital and femoral branches as it nears the inguinal ligament. The genital branch of the genitofemoral nerve passes through the deep inguinal ring, passing into the spermatic cord to supply the cremaster muscle. The femoral branch (L1 fibers only) of the genitofemoral nerve passes under the inguinal ligament medial to the psoas tendon, on the external iliac artery, and then pierces the fascia lata to supply sensation to a small area of skin in the region of the femoral triangle.

Lateral femoral cutaneous nerve

The lateral femoral cutaneous nerve is formed from the posterior divisions of L2 and 3 and emerges lateral to the psoas. It runs across the iliacus muscle, deep to the iliac fascia. Branches here supply the parietal peritoneum lining the iliac fossa. The lateral femoral cutaneous nerve then runs under the inguinal ligament – or sometimes pierces through it – about 1 cm medial to the anterior superior iliac spine. Separate anterior and posterior branches pierce the fascia lata to supply cutaneous sensation to the lateral thigh, from the greater trochanter to the knee.

Femoral nerve

The femoral nerve is formed from posterior divisions of L2, 3 and 4, and will therefore principally supply extensor muscles (of the knee). It emerges slightly lower down the lateral border of the psoas muscle, and stays close to this lateral border as it runs towards the inguinal ligament. It

gives branches to the iliacus muscle, then passes under the inguinal ligament, giving a branch to the pectineus. It then lies in the femoral triangle, lateral to the femoral artery in its sheath. Almost immediately upon its entrance into the thigh, the femoral nerve divides into spaghetti-like branches which supply the musculature of the anterior compartment of the thigh, the skin of the anterior and lower medial thigh, and the medial side of the leg and ankle (Figure 8.3.5).

Of these branches, the medial cutaneous femoral nerve runs medially across the femoral artery and vein, piercing the fascia lata mid thigh to supply the lower, medial side of the thigh. Two nerves supply the sartorius, and one of these pierces the muscle to continue as the intermediate cutaneous nerve of the thigh, supplying the skin of the anterior thigh down to the knee. Another two branches supply the rectus femoris, with one of these also supplying sensory twigs to the hip joint. A large branch, the nerve to the vastus medialis, runs down with the femoral artery into the adductor (or subsartorial) canal, to supply the vastus medialis and the knee joint. The nerves to the vastus lateralis and intermedius also supply the knee joint. One branch of the femoral nerve continues past the knee: the saphenous nerve runs into the subsartorial (adductor) canal, crossing from the lateral to the medial side of the femoral artery, and emerging posterior to the tendon of sartorius near the knee. It then joins the long saphenous vein and supplies the skin of the lateral aspect of the knee, leg and ankle (Figure 8.3.6).

105

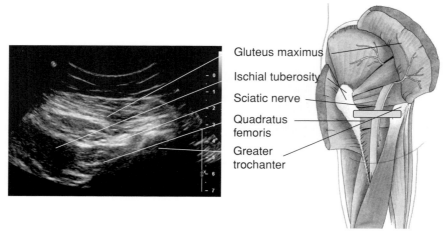

Gluteus maximus
Ischial tuberosity
Sciatic nerve
Quadratus femoris
Greater trochanter

Figure 8.3.6 Saphenous nerve.

Obturator nerve

The obturator nerve represents the anterior divisions of L2, 3 and 4 anterior primary rami, and supplies the adductors of the thigh. It is a much smaller nerve than the femoral, and emerges medial to the psoas muscle, crossing the pelvic brim and running anteriorly on the obturator internus muscle, supplying sensation to the pelvic parietal peritoneum. The obturator nerve converges with the obturator vessels on the upper part of the obturator foramen, through which it passes, splitting into anterior and posterior divisions. The anterior division runs over the obturator externus muscle, gives a twig to the hip joint, then runs down between the adductor longus and brevis, supplying both of these muscles and the gracilis, and giving off cutaneous branches via the subsartorial plexus. The posterior division of the obturator nerve pierces and supplies the obturator externus, and runs down into the thigh between the adductor brevis and magnus, supplying the latter and finally giving off a branch, which runs through the adductor hiatus, into the popliteal fossa to supply the knee joint.

The final branch of the lumbar plexus is the lumbosacral trunk. This also emerges medial to psoas and descends over the iliac ala into the true pelvis, carrying L4 and 5 fibers to reinforce the sacral plexus.

The sacral plexus

The sacral plexus is formed by the anterior primary rami of S1–S3, supplemented by the lumbosacral trunk, contributing L4 and L5 fibers. The tiny coccygeal plexus is formed by branches from S4, S5 and the coccygeal nerve, and supplies the skin over the coccyx.

The sacral plexus is formed within the pelvis, lying on piriformis muscle and beneath the parietal pelvic fascia and the internal iliac artery and its branches. Before the plexus forms, S1 and S2 branches are given off to supply the piriformis, and branches of S3 and S4 enter the pelvic surfaces of levator ani and coccygeus, supplying them. Pelvic splanchnic nerves leave S2, 3 and 4 roots, carrying parasympathetic fibers to the inferior hypogastric (pelvic) plexus, and thence to the pelvic viscera. The anterior primary rami then divide and reunite, forming the plexus itself. The branches of the sacral plexus leave the pelvis posteriorly, via the greater and lesser sciatic foramina (Figure 8.3.7).

The superior gluteal nerve (L4,5, S1) leaves the upper part of the sacral plexus, and passes out of the

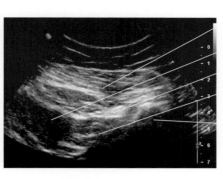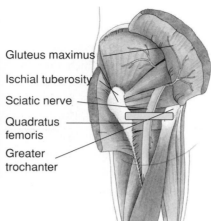

Gluteus maximus
Ischial tuberosity
Sciatic nerve
Quadratus femoris
Greater trochanter

Figure 8.3.7   Sciatic nerve.

pelvis through the greater sciatic foramen, emerging superior to the piriformis muscle in the buttock, to supply the gluteus medius and minimis, and tensor fasciae latae.

The inferior gluteal nerve (L5, S1,2) also passes through the greater sciatic foramen, but leaves beneath the piriformis, to supply the gluteus maximus. Neither gluteal nerve has any cutaneous distribution.

Sciatic nerve

The sciatic nerve (L4,5, S1,2,3) – by far the largest nerve of the sacral plexus – also emerges into the buttock inferior to the piriformis. It contains contributions from the anterior divisions of L4–S3 in its tibial part, and from the posterior divisions of L4–S2 in its common peroneal part.

In the buttock, the nerve to the quadratus femoris (L4,5, S1) lies deep to the sciatic nerve and the posterior femoral cutaneous nerve (S1,2,3) lies superficial to it. The nerve to the quadratus femoris sinks into that muscle to supply it, and also gives branches to the inferior gemellus and hip joint. The posterior femoral cutaneous nerve gives off a perineal branch to supply the posterior perineum, and gluteal branches supplying the skin of

the lower buttock. It then runs down the back of the thigh, superficial to the hamstrings and deep to the fascia lata, with branches supplying the skin of the posterior thigh and popliteal fossa (Figure 8.3.8, on DVD).

The nerve to the obturator internus (L5, S1,2) leaves the greater sciatic foramen beneath the piriformis and loops around the base of the ischial spine, lateral to the pudendal vessels, to run forwards on the sidewall of the ischioanal fossa and supply the obturator internus. It also supplies the superior gemellus muscle.

The pudendal nerve (S2,3,4) exits the pelvis through the greater sciatic foramen, below the piriformis muscle and very close to the ischial spine. It loops around the sacrospinous ligament, medial to the pudendal vessels, and re-enters the pelvis through the lesser sciatic foramen. It now lies below the levator ani and is in position to send branches to the perineum. The main nerve lies with the pudendal vessels in the pudendal (Alcock's) canal, in the fascia over the lower part of the obturator internus. Inferior rectal branches run medially to the external anal sphincter, mucosa of the lower anal canal, and anal skin. The pudendal nerve divides into its terminal branches, the

107

perineal nerve and dorsal nerve of the penis or clitoris, within the pudendal canal. As it approaches the ischial tuberosity, the perineal nerve gives off a posterior scrotal or labial nerve, which runs forward, superficial to the perineal membrane, to supply the skin of the posterior scrotum or labia majora. The perineal nerve itself, and the dorsal nerve of the penis or clitoris, run anteriorly, superior (deep) to the perineal membrane. The perineal nerve gives muscular branches to the perineal muscles and the sphincter urethrae, and sensory branches to the urethra. The dorsal nerve of the penis or clitoris pierces the perineal membrane just under the pubic symphysis and supplies the shaft and glans of the penis or clitoris.

The perforating cutaneous nerve (S2,3) perforates the sacrotuberous ligament and supplies the skin of the lower buttock.

The course and distribution of the sciatic nerve

The sciatic nerve emerges into the buttock through the greater sciatic foramen, beneath the piriformis and under cover of the gluteus maximus. It runs down over the obturator internus tendon and the gemelli, where it lies halfway between the ischial tuberosity and the greater trochanter of the femur, and passes into the thigh. It runs straight down the back of the thigh, passing under the long head of the biceps femoris, and over the underlying adductor magnus to lie between the two hamstring groups. The tibial component of the greater sciatic nerve supplies the hamstrings in the thigh, as well as the hamstring part of the adductor magnus, i.e. that part of the muscle arising from the ischium.

The sciatic nerve usually divides into tibial and common peroneal nerves in mid thigh, but this is subject to anatomical variation. The split can occur higher up the thigh. Sometimes the two nerves even emerge separately in the buttock, with the common peroneal nerve piercing the piriformis and the tibial nerve emerging below it.

The tibial component of the common peroneal nerve supplies the long head of the biceps femoris, semimembranosus and semitendinosus, and the hamstring part of adductor magnus (attaching to the ischium). The short head of the biceps femoris is supplied by the common peroneal component of the sciatic nerve.

Popliteal fossa

The tibial nerve emerges at the upper apex of the diamond-shaped popliteal fossa, between the diverging hamstrings, and runs straight down to its lower apex, created by the converging bellies of the gastrocnemius muscle. In the popliteal fossa, it lies superficial to the deeper popliteal vein and artery, and gives three genicular branches to the knee joint, muscular branches to the popliteus, both heads of the gastrocnemius, the soleus and the plantaris, and gives off the cutaneous sural nerve (Figure 8.3.9). The sural nerve runs down the groove between the two heads of the gastrocnemius and pierces the deep fascia midway down the calf to become superficial. Then the sural nerve joins with the sural communicating nerve to lie lateral to the short saphenous vein. It supplies the postero-lateral aspect of the calf and ankle, running anterior to the lateral malleolus to supply the lateral side of the foot along to the little toe. The tibial nerve leaves the popliteal fossa by passing deep to the converging heads of the gastrocnemius, and diving under the fibrous arch of soleus to lie between the superficial and deep groups of calf muscles, supplying both groups. It then runs down to the ankle with the posterior tibial artery. At the ankle, it passes midway between the medial malleolus and tendo calcaneus, lying between the posterior tibial artery (anteriorly) and the tendon of the flexor hallucis longus (posteriorly). As it passes under the flexor retinaculum, it divides into its terminal branches: the medial and lateral plantar nerves, which wrap around the medial arch of the foot to pass into the sole and

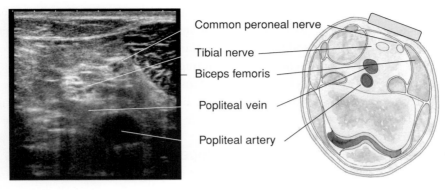

Common peroneal nerve
Tibial nerve
Biceps femoris
Popliteal vein
Popliteal artery

Figure 8.3.9 Popliteal fossa.

supply the instrinsic muscles of the foot, and the skin of the sole.

Tibial nerve

The common peroneal nerve emerges to lie lateral in the popliteal fossa, hugging the medial border of the biceps femoris and running anteriorly to disappear into the substance of peroneus longus, where it lies against the neck of the fibula. In the popliteal fossa, it gives off the sural communicating nerve, and the lateral cutaneous nerve of the calf (supplying the upper, lateral part of the calf). It also provides superior and inferior genicular nerves, and the recurrent genicular nerve, which supplies the superior tibiofibular joint as well as the knee. Within the peroneus longus muscle, the common peroneal nerve divides into deep and superficial parts. The superficial peroneal nerve supplies the peroneus longus and brevis in the lateral compartment of the leg, then emerges anterior to the tendon of the peroneus longus as medial and lateral branches which run over the dorsum of the foot to the toes, supplying most of the skin in this area. The deep peroneal nerve spirals around the fibula, to run onto the anterior surface of the interosseous membrane, lying with the anterior tibial vessels between the extensor digitorum longus and the tibialis anterior. It supplies the muscles of the anterior compartment: the tibialis anterior, the extensor hallucis, the

extensor digitorum longus, and the peroneus tertius. It then runs with the dorsalis pedis artery, on its medial side, across the extensor digitorum brevis, which it supplies, and emerges to become superficial between the large and the second toe, supplying the skin of the first toe cleft (Figure 8.3.10, on DVD).

Part 4: Ultrasound-guided approaches for the upper limb

Introduction

The key step for successful regional anesthetic blocks is the optimal distribution of local anesthetics around the nerve structures. Therefore it is important to position the needle tip close to the nerve without damaging neural structures. This is made possible by using ultrasound guidance. The Vienna scientific study group has shown, during the past decade, that ultrasound can be used for almost all regional anesthetic techniques to significantly improve the quality of the block. In addition, by using ultrasound guidance, complications such as intraneuronal injection or intravascular injection of local anesthetic can be avoided. However, before ultrasound can be used in daily clinical practice, some form of structured education of anesthetists in this technique needs to be undertaken. This education includes a detailed anatomical knowledge of the structures involved; the physics of ultrasound and the characteristics of the equipment; image capture and optimization; and the needling techniques appropriate to regional anesthesia. In addition, the availability of appropriate ultrasound equipment with a combination of suitable probes is essential.

In the past three years our study group has performed over 4000 blocks under ultrasonographic guidance with a success rate in excess of 98%. Not only has the success rate increased rapidly compared with conventional nerve stimulator techniques, but also the sensory and motor onset times for all the blocks has improved significantly.

Sonographic appearances of the brachial plexus

The sonographic character of the brachial plexus has been described either as hypoechoic or hyperechoic. There are several factors that influence the ultrasonographic image of a nerve such as the size of the nerve, the frequency used and the angle of incidence of the ultrasound beam. In the transverse view (cross-section), which is the common scanning view used to perform most of the blocks, nerves are visualized as multiple round or oval hypoechoic areas encircled by a relative hyperechoic outer layer or covering. These hypoechoic structures represent the fascicles of the nerves, while the hyperechoic background reflects the connective tissue between neuronal structures. In a longitudinal view, nerves appear as a relatively hyperechoic band characterized by multiple discontinuous hypoechoic stripes which are separated by hypoechoic lines. As the fascicles are the main sonographic features of peripheral nerves, it has been termed a "fascicular pattern", in contrast to tendons, which are represented as a "fibrillar pattern" with multiple hyperechoic continuous lines. The number of fascicles shown with ultrasound does not represent the true number of fascicles within the nerve, as the very small fascicles cannot be identified with ultrasound. While the fascicular pattern seems to be typical for large peripheral nerves (e.g.

median, ulna and radial nerves), it is not the same for smaller nerves such as the recurrent laryngeal or the vagal nerves (appearing hypoechoic – dark throughout).

Most of the peripheral nerves in the upper limb can be seen using ultrasound throughout their entire course, unless obscured by bone or vessels.

Upper extremity nerve blocks

The brachial plexus is formed by the anterior parts of the roots C5–T1. The formation of the brachial plexus includes C4 in 60% of cases and T2 in 30% of cases. The roots pass dorsal to the vertebral artery through the intervertebral foramina. As the roots leave the foramina, they immediately enter the interscalene space. Within this space, the roots descend towards the first rib and converge to form the three trunks (superior, medial, and inferior). At the supraclavicular level, each of the three trunks divides into an anterior and posterior division. After the trunks have crossed the first rib, at the level of the upper border of the clavicle, they subdivide into three cords (posterior, lateral, and medial), from which the terminal nerves are derived. At the level of the first rib, the cords of the brachial plexus rotate around the subclavian artery like a corkscrew, so that directly below the clavicle, the lateral cord is anterior and medial to the posterior cord. At this level, the medial cord is below the lateral cord. The position nomenclature of the cords is only valid at the axillary level (see below).

Interscalene brachial plexus block

The indication for the interscalene brachial plexus block is surgical procedures at the level of the shoulder and the upper arm. The technique was described initially by Winnie [1] using a puncture site at the posterior border of the sternocleidomastoid muscle at the level of the cricoid cartilage. The needle was introduced in a perpendicular direction to the skin. This technique was modified by Meier et al. [2] to a more cranial level of puncture and a more tangential needle direction. The perpendicular needle direction has been associated with an increased incidence of complications, including epidural and intrathecal placement of local anesthetic leading to bilateral block and total spinal; and vertebral artery puncture, inadvertent intravascular injection into the vertebral artery resulting in seizures.

The brachial plexus can be easily visualized by ultrasound at this level. A preliminary scan of the area starts at the level of the larynx, where the thyroid gland and the carotid artery as well as the internal jugular vein are visible. It is possible to visualize the vagal nerve between these two vessels (Figure 8.4.1, on DVD).

By moving the probe laterally, the lateral border of the sternocleidomastoid muscle is identified. Posterior to this, the scalenus anterior muscle and scalenus medius muscle are seen. With a slight caudal angulation of the probe the nerve structure of the brachial plexus roots is visualized in a transverse view as multiple round or oval hypoechoic areas between the anterior and median scalene muscles (Figure 8.4.2, on DVD).

It is important to realize that the diameter of the roots and the characteristic of the image of the nerve structures shows a high degree of variability between individuals. Even the position of the interscalene groove is not always at the lateral border of the sternocleidomastoid muscle. The groove itself may be either underneath or anterior to the lateral border of the sternocleidomastoid muscle. The appearance of the roots is dependent on the anisotropic behavior of nerve structures. In other words, based on the fact that not all the roots are running parallel to each other, it is not possible to visualize all the five roots with one probe position because the sound beam will be reflected off some of the roots and deflected by others. The result is that only two or three roots are usually visible in the same scanning plane. Tissue contrast of the connective tissue, fat and muscles may influence the quality of the picture seen, increasing the individual variability seen.

The nerve roots can be seen exiting the intervertebral foramen and entering the interscalene space by focusing on the transverse processes. The highest level of the brachial plexus is the C5 root, which appears between the transverse processes of C5 and C6. At this level, the visualization of only one root is possible. By shifting the scanning head downwards the C6 root will appear under the transverse process of C6. With a further shift, we will find the C5 to C7 roots within the interscalene space. Even smaller nerves can be seen with the higher specification machines and the origin of the long thoracic nerve may be identified (Figure 8.4.3, on DVD).

By shifting the scanning head further downwards the C8 and T1 roots will be visualized, commonly close to the pleura and the subclavian artery. It is necessary to identify the brachial plexus and to consider the best course of the needle through the tissues avoiding large blood vessels before an ultrasound-guided interscalene block is performed.

The endpoint for the needle is not the nerve roots per se, which may lead to pain and damage, but the connective tissue lateral of the roots to enable local anesthetic spread around the roots. Following puncture of the skin 1 cm cranial to the probe, a 5 cm 22 g needle (facetted tip) is placed in the interscalene space, at the level of C5 or C6. This procedure can either be performed using an in-plane or out-of-plane technique as described previously. Injection of 10–15 ml local anesthetic is usually sufficient for shoulder surgery. This volume is not sufficient to reliably block the lower root (C8–T1). If anesthesia of the elbow or medial part of the forearm is required then the needle should be repositioned towards the lower roots and further local anesthetic injected at this level (Figure 8.4.4 and Figure 8.4.5).

For continuous interscalene plexus anesthesia a catheter is placed in the interscalene space.

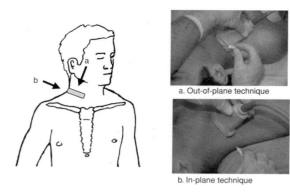

a. Out-of-plane technique

b. In-plane technique

Figure 8.4.4 Interscalene brachial plexus, block position and techniques.

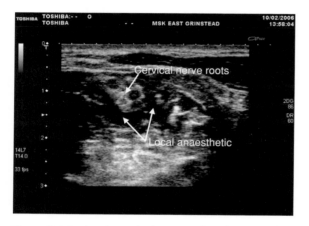

Figure 8.4.5 Local anesthetic surrounding the cervical roots in the interscalene groove.

Supraclavicular brachial plexus block

The supraclavicular block is one of the oldest approaches for anesthetising the brachial plexus (Kulenkampff, 1911) and at this level the trunks and divisions are tightly packed and lie on the first rib posterior to the subclavian artery. The main disadvantage of this technique has always been the close proximity of the pleura and the risk of inadvertent puncture leading to a pneumothorax. The indications for this approach are all surgery on the arm, forearm and hand, and pain relief. However, this technique does not reliably block the lower trunk and is prone to "miss" the ulnar side of the hand.

In 1994 the Vienna study group developed an ultrasound-guided supraclavicular approach and compared this technique with the axillary approach. We demonstrated that both visualization and blockade of the brachial plexus was possible using ultrasound guidance, and this has also been confirmed by Williams *et al.* [3].

The entire brachial plexus can be visualized near the subclavian artery by placing the ultrasound probe in the supraclavicular fossa. Because the anatomical structures of interest are close to the skin, the best results can be achieved by using a high-frequency linear probe (10–14 MHz).

Figure 8.4.6 (on DVD) is a cross-section US view of supraclavicular fossa showing subclavian artery (SA), brachial plexus (BP), first rib (1R) and the cervical pleura (P).

At this level, the transformation of the roots into trunks is seen, and the presence of the transverse cervical artery can be noted. This artery, which is present in 60% of people, always crosses through the roots and trunks of the brachial plexus between the middle and lower trunk or between the C7 and C8 roots.

In some patients (frequently obese patients), the C8 and T1 roots are close to the pleura and will be seen behind and beside the subclavian artery. At this level, the trunks of the brachial plexus are extremely closely packed, and exact identification of the individual trunks, anterior and posterior divisions on a single picture is difficult. In practice, if the probe is moved slowly in a craniocaudal direction, it is possible to identify individual structures of the brachial plexus at this level.

The needle is introduced under the posterior border of the probe using an in-plane approach and directed, under direct vision, to the postero-lateral border of the subclavian artery. At this position the needle will be within the brachial plexus near the inferior trunk. An injection here of 10–15 ml of local anesthetic will block the brachial plexus (Figure 8.4.7).

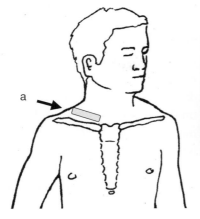
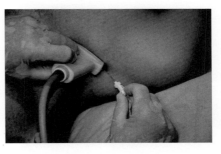

a. In-plane technique

Figure 8.4.7   Supraclavicular brachial plexus block, position and technique.

The supraclavicular approach is an excellent technique for brachial plexus block using ultrasound, as structures of interest are very superficial and excellent images can be easily achieved in all patients.

Infraclavicular brachial plexus block

The vertical infraclavicular brachial plexus block (VIB), initially described by Kilka *et al.* [4], is one of the most popular approaches to the brachial plexus. It provides a success rate between 88 and 95% with easily identified anatomical landmarks. Serious complications have been described with the VIB, if the puncture site is not accurately located and the needle direction is too medial. Greher *et al.* [5] investigated the reliability of the VIB point using ultrasound, and calculated a formula which resulted in a modification of the VIB point. The result of this ultrasonographic study showed that the predicted VIB point and the ultrasonographic-determined infraclavicular puncture site corresponded in less than 20% of cases. Neuburger *et al.* [6] confirmed these results in a clinical study, and corrected the former VIB point following the recommendations of Greher *et al.* [5]. He stated that "When the distance from jugular notch to acromion is less than 22 cm, for every cm less, the puncture site should be moved 2 mm laterally and for every cm greater than 22 cm the puncture site should be moved 2 mm medially."

As a consequence of these findings, it could be argued that all infraclavicular brachial plexus blocks should be performed under ultrasound guidance. To avoid inadvertent puncture of the cervical pleura, a more lateral approach can be used. The lateral infraclavicular brachial plexus block, initially described by Kapral *et al.* [7], is a safe alternative to the axillary approach giving a more consistent blockade of associated musculocutaneous, thoracodorsal, axillary and medial brachial cutaneous nerves.

The ultrasonographic findings of the infraclavicular part of the brachial plexus are not easy to understand, as the anatomical findings immediately under the clavicle are completely different compared to the findings more lateral under the coracoid process.

The brachial plexus passes over the first rib, beneath the clavicle passing into the apex of the axilla. After passing under the clavicle, the subclavian artery becomes the axillary artery. The three cords are positioned lateral to the artery and the subclavian vein is medial to the artery (Figure 8.4.8).

On entering the axilla, the cords of the plexus start to encircle the axillary artery. At the level

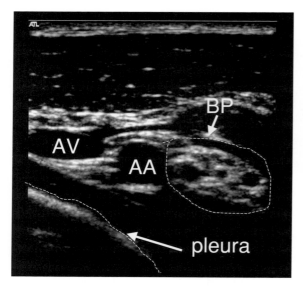

Figure 8.4.8 US view of the infraclavicular region (medial) showing the relationship of the brachial plexus to the axillary artery and vein (AA and AV) and pleura.

of the coracoid process and behind the pectoralis muscle, the cords lie in their true anatomical position in relation to the second part of the axillary artery; lateral cord – lateral to the artery; medial cord – medial to the artery; and posterior cord – posterior to the artery. Figure 8.4.9 (on DVD) shows the US view lateral infraclavicular region showing the relationship of the of the cords, medial cord (MC), lateral cord (LC), posterior cord (PC) to the axillary artery (AR).

In addition, the brachial plexus also now divides into its terminal branches. The major ones are the lateral cord which gives rise to the musculocutaneous and lateral root of the median nerve; the posterior cord gives rise to the axillary and radial nerve and the medial cord gives rise to the ulnar nerve and lateral root of the median nerve. Under perfect scanning conditions is possible to visualize most of these anatomical changes in detail.

Place the US probe underneath the clavicle with the long axis of the probe parallel to the clavicle to identify the brachial plexus lateral to the axillary artery.

Medial infraclavicular block position and technique (Figure 8.4.10, on DVD)

The needle is introduced in an out-of-plane approach above (cranial to) the probe [7]. The point of needle insertion is very close to the standard VIB insertion point, but ultimately depends on the ultrasound image and not on the measurements from the clavicle. The direction of the needle is nearly perpendicular to the skin. The image shows the brachial plexus lateral to the vessels and more lateral to the pleura. In clinical practice we prefer to insert the needle slightly lateral to the bundle of the three cords. Under direct vision, 20 ml of local anesthetic is injected as a single shot. The risk of pneumothorax, which has been described for the blind technique, is minimized and the success rate can be increased to close to 98–99%.

An alternative in-plane approach is achieved by inserting the needle under the lateral border of the probe. The needle is advanced according to the sonographic findings in an approximately 45° angle to the skin. The more lateral point of needle insertion might contribute to reduce the risk of complication, because with this approach the distance to the pleura is significantly increased. The endpoint of the needle insertion is lateral to the three cords, which is the same point as with the first technique.

With the probe in the parasagittal plane at the level of the coracoid process, two more recent techniques have been described by Klaastad and Sandhu. Klaastad used a linear probe 8–13 MHz, and Sandhu and Capal [8] used a curvilinear probe 2–5 MHz. At this level the individual cords are not easily seen, but the artery and vein are easily distinguished and the pleura does not represent a risk here, as it is more medial. The cords at this level surround the artery and the basis of this technique is a peri-arterial injection to ensure spread of local anesthetic around the artery.

The needle is inserted in an in-plane technique above the probe, either just beneath the coracoid process or just medal to it. The arm is slightly abducted to improve visualization of the cords and vessels. The needle is positioned close to the posterior border of the artery and 20 ml of local anesthetic is injected. Spread of local anesthetic should encircle the artery; if this does not happen, then the needle is repositioned anterior to the artery between the artery and vein (Figure 8.4.11, on DVD: lateral infraclavicular block position and technique. Figure 8.4.12, on DVD: cords of the brachial plexus with local anesthetic spread).

Axillary brachial plexus block

The axillary approach to the brachial plexus is still the most popular approach, due to the ease of performance and low incidence of side effects and complications. Despite this, Stark [9] reported three cases of permanent neurological damage following axillary brachial plexus anesthesia. The literature suggests that routine success rates can be as low as 70–80%. A possible reason for these unacceptably low success rates could be that using a puncture site above the axillary artery may result in failure to block the radial nerve [10]. Thus, despite the fact that the axillary brachial plexus block is extremely popular, many questions still remain.

Retzl et al. [11] showed that ultrasound can be used to identify nerves at the axillary level. The authors of that study described that the main nerves of the brachial plexus show several variations with regard to the axillary artery. In addition, the position of the nerves in relation to the axillary artery changes significantly even when light pressure is applied, such as during palpation of the axillary artery. These findings could also contribute to the high failure rate of axillary brachial plexus blocks.

The median nerve can be easily seen directly beside (lateral and above) the axillary artery. This nerve keeps its close position to the artery down to the level of the antecubital fossa, only changing its relationship from lateral to medial at some point. The ulnar nerve is medial (below) the artery, often beneath the axillary vein, and very superficial. It keeps this superficial position down to the level of the proximal forearm. The radial nerve that is sometimes the "problem nerve" during axillary plexus block [12] can be identified below the artery. Figure 8.4.13 (on DVD) is a cross-sectional US view of the axilla showing axillary artery (AA), axillary vein (AV), biceps muscle (B), coracobrachialis muscle (CB), triceps muscle (T), median nerve (M), ulnar nerve (U), radial nerve (R), and musculocutaneous nerve (MSC).

With the probe placed transversely across the axilla just below the level of the insertion of the pectoralis major muscles (anterior axillary fold), identify the axillary artery, vein(s) and nerves. Using either an in-plane or out-of-plane technique, a needle is inserted either above (lateral to) or below (medial to) the artery and placed close to each of the median, ulnar and radial nerves. Local anesthetic (5–8 ml) is usually sufficient to ensure spread around and blockade of each nerve.

The axillary technique is similar to the peripheral stimulation technique, which is essentially a multi-injection technique as described by Koscielnak-Nielsen et al. [13] and Fanelli et al. [12]. In about 10% of the cases, the presence of the septal fascial can be identified between the nerves using ultrasound, which may impair spread of the local anesthetic. Their presence has often been denied in the literature [14] (Figures 8.4.14 and 8.4.15, both on DVD).

The musculocutaneous nerve at this level is separate from the other nerves and lies between the biceps and coracobrachialis muscles, in most cases. So this nerve is not reliably blocked by the axillary approach and may need to be injected separately. Usually the identification of the musculocutaneous nerve by ultrasound is easy and the blockade can be performed with 3–5 ml of local anesthetic by a slight movement of the needle in a lateral direction (Figure 8.4.16, on DVD: cross-sectional US view of musculocutaneous muscle. Figure 8.4.17, on DVD: musculocutaneous nerve block position and technique. Figure 8.4.18, on DVD: musculocutaneous nerve surrounded by local anesthetic).

Terminal peripheral nerves, radial, median and ulnar

The blockade of the terminal peripheral nerves of the upper limb is frequently used to top up more proximal approaches (failed blocks) or for post-operative analgesia. Classically, the techniques are performed using bony landmarks and have a high success rate.

With ultrasound it is possible to follow the path of all the peripheral nerves from the axilla to the elbow easily and then in the case of the ulnar and median to the wrist. The radial nerve divides close to the elbow and its deep branch is difficult to follow. The superficial radial nerve is very small and not easily seen. It is possible to block all the peripheral nerves at many places in the arm and forearm.

Radial nerve block

The nerve is best approached either in the mid-humeral position or just above the elbow, three fingers breadth above the lateral epicondyle of the humerus. At these two sites the radial nerve is easily to identify (Figure 8.19, on DVD: cross-sectional US view of the lower arm, showing humerus (H), radial nerve (R) within triceps muscle (T)).

In the midhumeral approach, the radial nerve is positioned in the radial groove of the humerus. Proximal to the groove, the nerve can be identified in a bundle together with the profunda brachii artery. This artery accompanies the nerve in 50% of patients. Using a short axis technique, the needle can be positioned close to the nerve and 3–5 ml of local anesthetic injected.

Above the elbow, the radial nerve can be seen passing around the humerus, between the two heads of triceps, emerging at the elbow between brachialis and brachioradialis. It can be identified proximally before it divides into its superficial and deep branches. Using either an in-plane or out-of-plane approach, the needle is positioned close to the nerve and 3–5 ml of local anesthetic injected (Figure 8.4.20, on DVD: radial nerve block position and technique).

Median nerve block

At the level of the elbow, the median nerve lies medial to, and slightly deeper than, the brachial artery. Using either an in-plane or out-of-plane technique, position the needle close to the nerve and inject 3–5 ml of local anesthetic (Figure 8.4.21, on DVD: cross-sectional US view at the elbow showing brachial artery (BA) and the median nerve (M); Figure 8.4.22, on DVD: median nerve block (elbow) – positioning and technique; Figure 8.4.23, on DVD: median nerve surrounded by local anesthetic).

At the level of the wrist, the median nerve is very superficial (less than 0.5 cm from the skin) and easily seen between the tendons of flexor carpi radialis and palmaris longus, which is absent in 30% of people. The needle is inserted in an in-plane technique at the level of the proximal wrist crease. Position the needle next to the nerve and inject 2–5 ml of local anesthetic (Figure 8.4.24, on DVD: median nerve longitudinal view – forearm; Figure 8.4.25, on DVD: cross-sectional US view at level of the wrist, showing flexor carpi radialis (FCR), median nerve (M), tendons of the flexor digitorum superficialis and profunda (FDS and FDP); Figure 8.4.26, on DVD: median nerve block (wrist) position and technique; Figure 8.4.27, on DVD: median nerve surrounded by local anesthetic).

Ulnar nerve block

Blocking the ulnar nerve close to the elbow had some proven disadvantages when performed either blindly or with a nerve stimulator technique. The success rate may be very low – 50–80% – and cases of ulna nerve damage or neuritis have been described. These two drawbacks may be explained by the presence of intramuscular membranes (flexor carpi ulnaris) close to the ulnar nerve, either by restricting the spread of local anesthetic or by causing high injection pressures. Two different approaches can be used for the ulnar nerve, either 10–15 cm above (proximal) the ulnar sulcus or 10–15 cm below (distal) the ulnar sulcus.

In the proximal technique the ulnar nerve can be seen subcutaneously in the medial side of the upper arm. Using either an in-plane or out-of-plane technique, the needle is positioned close to the nerve and 3–5 ml of local anesthetic is injected.

In the distal technique, the nerve is seen on the medial side of the forearm beneath the flexor carpi ulnaris accompanied by the ulnar artery. Using either an in-plane or out-of-plane technique, the needle is positioned close to the nerve and 3–5 ml of local anesthetic is injected (Figure 8.4.28, on DVD: cross-sectional US view of the forearm showing the flexor carpi ulnaris (FCU), ulnar artery (UA) and the ulnar nerve (U); Figure 8.4.29, on DVD: ulnar nerve block position and technique; Figure 8.4.30, on DVD: ulnar nerve surrounded by local anesthetic).

REFERENCES

1. Winnie AP. The interscalene brachial plexus block. *Anesthesia and Analgesia* 1970;49: 455–66.

2. Meier G, Bauereis C, Maurer H, Meier T. Interscalenare Plexusblockade: anatomische Voraussetzungen – anasthesiologische und operative Aspekte. *Anaesthesist* 2001;50: 333–41.

3. Williams SR, Chovinard P, Arcand G, *et al.* Ultrasound guidance speeds execution and improves the quality of supraclavicular block. *Anesthesia and Analgesia* 2003;97:1518–23.

4. Kilka HG, Geiger P, Mehrkens HH. Infraclavicular plexus blockade. A new method for anaesthesia of the upper extremity. An anatomical and clinical study. *Anaesthetist* 1995;44:339–44.

5. Greher M, Retzl G, Niel P, Kamholz L, Marhofer P, Kapral S. Ultrasonographic assessment of topographic anatomy in volunteers suggest a modification of the infraclavicular vertical brachial block. *British Journal of Anaesthesia* 2002;88:632–6.

6. Neuburger M, Kaiser H, Rembold-Schuster I, Landes H. Vertical infraclavicular brachial–plexus blockade. A clinical study of reliability of a new method for plexus anesthesia of the upper extremity. *Anaesthetist* 1998;47:595–9.

7. Kapral S, Jandrasits O, Schabernig C, *et al.* Lateral infraclavicular plexus block vs. axillary block for hand and forearm surgery. *Acta Anaesthesiologica Scandinavica* 1999;43: 1047–52.

8. Sandhu NS, Capal LM. Ultrasound-guided infraclavicular brachial plexus block. *British Journal of Anaesthesia* 2002;89:254–9.

9. Stark RH. Neurological injury from axillary block anesthesia. *Journal of Hand Surgery* 1996;21:391–6.

10. Meier G, Maurer H, Bauereis C. Axillary brachial plexus block. Anatomical investigations to improve radial nerve block. *Anaesthetist* 2003;52:535–9.

11. Retzl G, Kapral S, Greher M, Mauritz W. Ultrasonographic findings of the axillary part of the brachial plexus. *Anesthesia and Analgesia* 2001;92:1271–5.

12. Fanelli G, Casati A, Beccaria P, Cappelleri G, Albertin A, Torri G. Interscalene brachial plexus anaesthesia with small volumes of ropivacaine 0.75%: effects of the injection technique on the onset time of nerve blockade. *European Journal of Anaesthesiology* 2001;18:54–8.

13. Koscielnak-Nielsen ZJ, Stens-Pedersen HL, Lippert FK. Readiness for surgery after axillary

block: single or multiple injection techniques. *European Journal of Anaesthesiology* 1997;14: 164-71.

14. Thompson GE, Rorie DK. Functional anatomy of the brachial plexus sheath. *Anesthesiology* 1983;59:117-22.

FURTHER READING

De Andres J, Sala-Blanch X. Ultrasound in the practice of brachial plexus anesthesia. *Regional Anesthesia Pain Medicine* 2002;27:77-89.

Fleischmann E, Marhofer P, Greher M, Waltl B, Sitzwohl C, Kapral S. Brachial plexus anaesthesia in children: lateral infraclavicular vs. axillary approach. *Paediatric Anaesthesia* 2003;13:103-8.

Kapral S, Krafft P, Eibenberger K, Fitzgerald R, Gosch M, Weinstabl C. Ultrasound-guided supraclavicular approach for regional anesthesia of the brachial plexus. *Anesthesia and Analgesia* 1994;78:507-13.

La Grange P, Foster PA, Pretorius LK. Application of the Doppler ultrasound blood flow detector in supraclavicular brachial plexus block. *British Journal of Anaesthesia* 1978;50:965-7.

Perlas A, Chan VWS, Simons M. Brachial plexus examination and localization using ultrasound and electrical stimulation; a volunteer study. *Anesthesiology* 2003;99:429-35.

Peterson MK. Ultrasound-guided nerve blocks. *British Journal of Anaesthesia* 2002;88:621-4.

Part 5: Ultrasound-guided techniques for lower limb blocks

Introduction

Peripheral nerve blocks offer an excellent addition or an alternative to general anesthesia for surgical procedures on the lower limb, particularly for older and cardiovascularly compromised patients. The introduction of newer and more effective anticoagulation drugs such as low molecular weight heparins (LMWHs), direct oral thrombin inhibitors, platelet ADP receptor antagonists and glycoprotein IIb/IIIa receptor inhibitors may lead to an increased risk of bleeding and hematoma when neuraxial blocks (spinal, epidural) are performed. In these cases, regional anesthesia provides a safer alternative. Guidelines for neuraxial anesthesia in these patients are published [1]. In trauma care or when emergency surgery is necessary, a detailed drug history may not be forthcoming, and in these cases postponement of the surgical procedure is often not possible. Therefore it is important to have available reliable techniques to block the peripheral nerves of the lumbosacral plexus for the safe perioperative management of these patients.

It is important to note that some of the techniques using ultrasound are commonly described in the literature, and some are the authors' personal experience and are still under investigation. All techniques described are used in routine clinical practice by the authors.

Posterior lumbar plexus block (psoas compartment)

The lumbar plexus is derived from the anterior rami of the L1-4 roots. After exiting the intervertebral foramina, the nerves form the lumbar plexus within the body of the psoas muscle, comprising of: the iliohypogastric nerve (T12, L1), the ilioinguinal nerve (L1), the genitofemoral nerve (L1,2), the lateral femoral cutaneous nerve (L2,3), the femoral nerve (L1-4) and the obturator nerve (L2-4). It was previously assumed that the lumbar plexus and its branches are located within a potential space between the psoas major and quadratus lumborum muscles, the so-called psoas compartment [2]. Actually, this topographical situation occurs only in rare cases [3]. In the majority, the lumbar plexus is situated within the substance of the psoas major muscle [3-6].

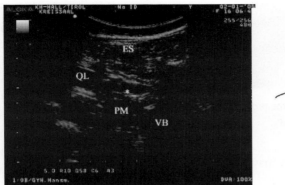
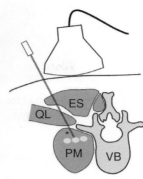

Figure 8.5.2 Cross-sectional view of the lumbar plexus at the level of L3, where the * indicates the nerve root between the posterior and middle third of the psoas major muscle (PM) (ES: erector spinae muscle, QL: quadratus lumborum muscle, VB: vertebral body).

The concept of the psoas compartment block is to place the needle within the lumbar plexus by means of a paravertebral approach at the level L4–5 [2]. Techniques used to identify this space or plexus have included loss of resistance [2], elicitation of paresthesia [7] and nerve stimulation [8]. These "blind" techniques may fail [9], as the psoas compartment block represents a deep block with skin–plexus distances occasionally exceeding 8 cm in obese individuals [5, 10].

For the ultrasound-guided approach to the psoas compartment, the patient can be positioned either prone, with a cushion placed under the abdomen to reduce lumbar lordosis, or in the lateral decubitus position with the hips flexed. A curvilinear 2–5 MHz probe provides good tissue penetration and gives an excellent overview of the lumbar paravertebral region [10]. In children and infants, higher frequencies are used [11].

In a longitudinal paravertebral plane, the echoes of the transverse processes are counted beginning at the sacrum (Figure 8.5.1 (on DVD): longitudinal US view of lumbar region).

Identify the L3–4 and L4–5 levels; both are suitable for an ultrasound-guided approach. At the level L4–5, sonography may be impaired in male patients due to tall iliac crests which cause bony shadowing. The lumbar paravertebral region is best visualized in a transverse plane at midway between the transverse processes of L3–4 or L4–5. The following structures need to be seen clearly on the scan: the erector spinae, the quadratus lumborum muscle, the psoas major muscle and, if possible, the lumbar plexus (Figure 8.5.2).

In children, sonographic identification of these structures is considerably easier and more reliable due to the shorter skin–nerve distance and their size [12]. This is not the case in many adults due to a greater skin–nerve distance and the limits of the axial and lateral resolution at such low ultrasound frequencies. Therefore the combined use of ultrasound with a nerve stimulator to elicit quadriceps muscle twitches for lumbar plexus location is advisable in adult patients. In young, slim adults the lumbar plexus can be clearly seen in some cases.

The needle is introduced approximately 4–5 cm lateral and parallel to the spinous processes in an in-plane approach and directed towards the posterior part of the psoas major muscle. The needle may be seen as a hyperechoic linear reflection [12]. After eliciting quadriceps muscle twitches and negative aspiration, 20 ml of local anesthetic is injected under ultrasound guidance (Figure 8.5.3).

Nerve stimulation is not necessary in children since direct visualization of the lumbar plexus is possible, and depending on the skin-plexus

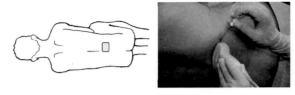

Figure 8.5.3 Lumbar plexus block. Position of the probe relative to the cannula using the in-line technique.

distances [11] a needle length of 50 mm may be appropriate in children under 12 years.

In summary, ultrasound guidance for posterior lumbar plexus block offers an alternative technique to the psoas compartment in children, but has significant limitations in adults and should only be considered by experienced ultrasound practitioners.

Ilioinguinal/iliohypogastric nerve block

The ilioinguinal/iliohypogastric nerve block is used for inguinal hernia repair and hydrocele surgery. The nerves arise from the roots of L1 or T12/L1 and lie in a variable position between the three abdominal muscles: external and internal oblique, and transversus abdominis [13]. The conventional technique is infiltration of 10–20 ml of local anesthetic into the abdominal wall, 1–2 cm medial to the superior anterior iliac spine [14]. Common side effects include transient quadriceps paresis [15] or femoral nerve palsy [16], and serious complications such as colonic puncture [17] and pelvic hematoma [18] have been reported. Despite using single or double "plop" techniques, depending on the depth of the puncture [19], the incidence of poor perioperative analgesia still lies between 20 and 30%.

Ultrasound guidance offers the possibility for the direct visualization of the nerves in relationship to the muscles of the abdominal wall. Figure 8.5.4 (on DVD) shows a transverse view of the ilioinguinal nerve medial to the superior anterior iliac spine using a high-frequency linear probe. An injection is performed with a 50 mm (80 mm in obese patients) needle (facetted tip), using either an in-plane or out-of-plane technique (Figure 8.5.5 (on DVD): ilioinguinal nerve block technique). After an initial injection of 0.5 ml of local anesthetic, 0.05–0.1 ml/kg (3–8 ml) is injected. It is important to observe the spread of local anesthetic during administration, because if the local anesthetic does not spread to the iliohypogastric nerve, the needle should be redirected.

Ultrasound-guided ilioinguinal/iliohypogastric nerve blocks have been scientifically evaluated in children, but not in adults. Preliminary results are encouraging in terms of clinical effectiveness and practicability of this technique. It is important to note that no correlations were found between weight and height to the distance from the nerves to the anterior superior iliac spine, or the depth of the nerves, or their distance to the peritoneum. In light of these findings, it is easy to see why all the above complications have been described.

Femoral nerve block

The commonest technique for femoral nerve block is Winnie's 3 : 1 block, used for surgical procedures of the anterior part of the thigh and knee down to the medial border of the ankle. This technique is described as blocking three nerves: femoral, lateral cutaneous nerve of thigh and obturator nerve with one single inguinal perivascular injection. Our group described this technique under ultrasound guidance in 1997 [20]. We observed significantly faster sensory onset times and improved quality of both sensory and motor block compared with the conventional nerve stimulator technique (Table 8.5.1). In addition, reduced volumes of local anesthetics provided an improved blockade [21]. This has particular advantages in patient in whom combined blocks (sciatic and femoral) may pose an increased risk of systemic toxicity [22].

The femoral nerve is easily seen distal to the inguinal ligament, lateral to the femoral artery

Table 8.5.1 Comparison between ultrasonographic- and nerve stimulator-guided 3-in-1 block [20] with 20 ml bupivacaine 0.5%

	Ultrasound-guided	Nerve stimulator-guided
Sensory onset time	16±14 min*	27±16 min*
Complete 3-in-1 block	95%	85%
No obturator nerve blocked	0%	5%
No block	5%	10%

*Significant difference $p < 0.05$.

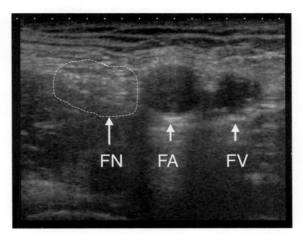

Figure 8.5.6   Cross-sectional view of the femoral nerve (FN) lateral the femoral vessels (FA and FV).

beneath iliacus fascia (Figure 8.5.6: cross-section US view of femoral nerve (FN) and femoral vessels (FA and FV)). A needle is inserted beneath the lateral border of the probe in an in-plane approach and positioned at the lateral aspect of the femoral nerve beneath the iliacus fascia (Figure 8.5.7). Ten milliliters of local anesthetic is injected for an isolated femoral nerve block, or 20 ml for a 3-in-1 block (Figure 8.5.8). It is possible to observe the spread, laterally and medially, of the local anesthetic beneath the fascia. It is not necessary to visualize the lateral cutaneous femoral and obturator nerves by ultrasound, as previous studies have proved the effectiveness of the single injection technique [20, 21]. In addition, both nerves are small. The anterior branch of the obturator nerve is located between the adductor longus and the adductor brevis, and a separate injection is needed to block this nerve as the distance from the entry point for the femoral nerve is too far. Blockade of all three nerves is seldom achieved with these volumes of local anesthetic. It is important to consider this technique at best a 2-in-1 block of femoral nerve and lateral cutaneous nerve of thigh, at worst a 1-in-1 femoral nerve block only.

Saphenous nerve block

In cases where only a sensory block of the femoral nerve is necessary for surgery in the region of the

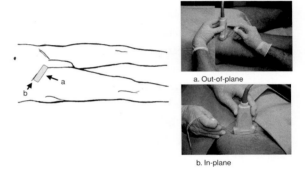

a. Out-of-plane

b. In-plane

Figure 8.5.7   Femoral nerve, technique.

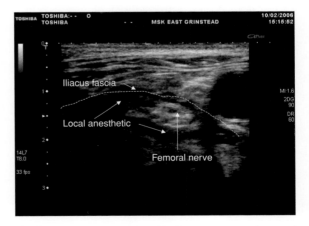

Figure 8.5.8   Femoral nerve block. Cross-sectional view of the femoral nerve (FN) with 10–20 ml local anesthetic (LA, black structure above the nerve) below the iliacus fascia.

121

median side of the lower leg down to the medial side of ankle and foot, a selective blockade of the saphenous nerve, the sensory end-branch of the femoral nerve, is appropriate. Conventional techniques are described as infiltration dorsal to the saphenous vein at the median side of the knee or slightly distal to the interarticular line [23]; trans-sartorial, or as a subcutaneous infiltration at the ankle [24]. The success rates of these blind techniques are low, between 45 and 60%, with a possible risk of nerve damage or hematoma [25]. Recently a stimulation technique for location of the saphenous nerve has been described [26].

Ultrasound is used to visualize the saphenous nerve in a cross-sectional view proximal to the knee in the subsartorial canal (adductor canal). Here it accompanies the nerve to the vastus medialis below the sartorius and gracilis muscles (Figure 8.5.9, on DVD). The site of injection should be selected where either the femoral artery is easily seen beneath sartorius in the adductor canal, or where the nerve emerges between the sartorius and the gracilis on the medial aspect of the lower thigh.

Using an in-plane technique, either place the needle within the canal next to the artery and inject to obtain a perivascular spread of local anesthetic, or position the needle close to the identified nerve within the subsartorial canal or between sartorius and gracilis and inject 5–10 ml of local anesthetic (Figure 8.5.10, on DVD: saphenous nerve block technique).

Infrapatellar branch

The infrapatellar branch of the saphenous nerve can be seen more distally. This sensory terminal branch of the saphenous leaves the main nerve to supply the medial border of the knee. The nerve can be selectively blocked with 1–2 ml of local anesthetic to help with pain control during and following knee arthroscopy [27] (Figure 8.5.11, on DVD: cross-section US view infrapatellar branch between showing the gracilis and the sartorius).

Sciatic nerve block

The sciatic nerve is formed by the sacral plexus (L4–S3). It is the largest nerve in the human body. The nerve can often be difficult to visualize clearly despite its size. This is in part due to the anisotropic nature of the nerve [28] and the attenuation of the ultrasound beam by the overlying muscles. The term "anisotropy" describes the sensitivity of the nerve to the angle of insonation, and highlights the importance of maintaining the probe and beam perpendicular to the nerve. In 1991, Graif *et al.* described the ultrasonographic appearance of the sciatic nerve, and referred to the possibility that beside the simple visualization of the nerve, an exact morphologic diagnosis is possible with ultrasound [29].

We perform three different approaches to the sciatic nerve: the subgluteal, midfemoral and popliteal approach. Blocks above the thigh (e.g. the Classical Labat approach) are difficult with ultrasound due to a relatively deep position of the nerve and large overlying muscle layers, which lead to poor ultrasonographic visualization of the target structure. From anatomical studies we know that the sciatic nerve is at its most superficial in the subgluteal region (immediately below the buttock crease).

Subgluteal approach

Ultrasonographic visualization of the sciatic nerve is easy at the subgluteal level where the nerve is located just below the buttock crease in the intramuscular groove between the long head of the biceps femoris muscle and the semitendinosus muscle midway in line with the mid point between the ischial tuberosity and the greater trochanter. A similar technique was described by Raj *et al.*, with the patient in a supine position and a success rate of 90% was achieved using 20 ml of local anesthetic [30].

At the subgluteal level, the sciatic nerve appears as an oval, hyperechoic structure with a transverse diameter up to 30 mm. It is appropriate in certain patients (e.g. obese) to use lower-frequency probes (curvilinear 2–5 MHz) for this approach, because the expected depth of the nerve may be greater than 5 cm (Figures 8.5.12 and 8.5.13, both on DVD).

This technique can be performed with the patient prone or in the lateral decubitus position depending on the patient's mobility (Figure 8.5.14). The needle is introduced using either an in-plane or out-of-plane technique and directed to lie close to the medial or lateral side of the nerve. Due to the size of the nerve, the needle may need to be positioned on both sides of the nerve to obtain an acceptable spread using 20 ml of local anesthetic.

Incomplete sciatic nerve blocks using nerve stimulator guidance may result from the fact that the sciatic nerve can divide into a tibial and a peroneal branch at the level of the piriformis muscle in 11% of patients [31]. Ultrasound guidance will allow the anesthetist to detect this situation and modify the procedure such that both branches are blocked effectively.

At the subgluteal level the posterior cutaneous nerve of the thigh is seen slightly medial and superficial to the sciatic nerve within the same muscle layer. A "blind" technique to block this nerve is described by Hughes and Brown. A needle is inserted beneath the superficial fascia at the medial border of the gluteus maximus muscle. Following a loss of resistance, 20 ml local anesthetic is injected. With ultrasound, if the posterior cutaneous nerve is seen to be anatomically distinct from the sciatic nerve it may be blocked separately, using 5–10 ml of local anesthetic (Figure 8.5.15).

Midthigh approach

One advantage of an ultrasound-guided peripheral nerve block is that a nerve can be blocked wherever it is seen. The sciatic nerve is exceptional, as it can be visualized throughout its entire path through the posterior thigh from the buttock to the popliteal fossa. Nevertheless, due to changes in the depth of

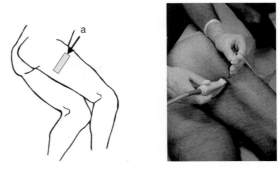

a. In-plane approach

Figure 8.5.14 Sciatic nerve, subgluteal technique.

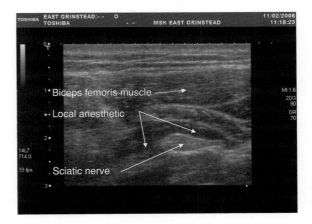

Figure 8.5.15 Sciatic nerve, showing local anesthetic spread.

the sciatic nerve and different overlying muscles, the quality of the images varies considerably.

Several approaches to the sciatic nerve within the thigh are described. Di Benedetto *et al.* describe an approach to the sciatic nerve 4 cm distal to a line drawn from the greater trochanter to the ischial tuberosity with a success rate of 94% [32]. The authors describe severe pain (12%) during performance of this block. More distal approaches have been described [33]; some of them involve a lateral approach [34]. Due to the lack of an easily palpable landmark within the thigh, all of these approaches are difficult to perform using peripheral nerve stimulation. With ultrasound, easy identification of the sciatic nerve can be performed at any level (Figure 8.5.16, on DVD: cross-section US view in midthigh and line drawing of technique).

The midthigh approach to the sciatic nerve is performed with the patient in a supine or lateral position. In most cases, an optimal ultrasonographic visualization of the nerve is possible between the proximal and middle third of the thigh, but once again blockade of the nerve will be performed wherever it is best seen. Injection of 10–20 ml of local anesthetic is usually sufficient.

Popliteal approach

The popliteal approach to the sciatic nerve is a popular regional anesthetic technique in children [35, 36] but also described in adults. The lateral popliteal approach has been shown to have advantages over the posterior approach in terms of sensory onset time and duration of sensory blockade [37]. The main disadvantage of a sciatic nerve block at the popliteal level is the inability to know the exact level at which the division of the tibial and peroneal components takes place. Ultrasound can accurately locate the level of this division [38].

Rivas Ferreira *et al.* described the use of ultrasound in combination with a nerve stimulator at the popliteal level via a posterior approach [39]. They suggest that the site of injection should be adjusted to ensure that it is just proximal to the division of the sciatic nerve. Failure to locate the nerve even with nerve stimulation has been reported by Sites *et al.* [40] in patients with diabetes, despite using currents of 2–4 mA. The subsequent successful use of ultrasound guidance in this small series of case reports supports our own observation that nerve stimulation may be ineffective in patients with neuropathies, lending further weight to the argument for the use of ultrasound in the clinical practice of (peripheral) regional anesthesia.

The popliteal nerve block is performed with the patient in the supine, prone or lateral positions, with the knee slightly flexed (Figures 8.5.17 and

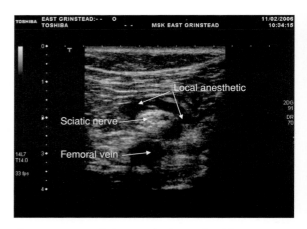

Figure 8.5.20 Sciatic nerve in the popliteal fossa, showing local anesthetic spread.

8.5.18, both on DVD). Following visualization of the sciatic nerve and its division, we choose an injection site either separate from the probe, laterally (in-plane approach through the biceps femoris muscle) or proximal/distal to the probe (out-of-plane approach) (Figure 8.5.19, on DVD: cross-section US view, with division of the sciatic nerve, tibial nerve (TN), common peroneal nerve (CPN), biceps femoris (BF) and popliteal vessels (PV and PA)).

Depending on the distribution of the local anesthetic, the needle may need to be repositioned to achieve complete circumferential spread of the local anesthetic. Injection of 10–20 ml of local anesthetic is sufficient in most patients, which is significantly lower compared with most of previous published techniques [41] (Figure 8.5.20).

Rectus sheath block

One common regional technique used but not described elsewhere is the rectus sheath block. This is not a block of nerves from the lumbosacral plexus, but due to its inherent simplicity deserves a mention here.

The rectus sheath block is a fascial plane block of the anterior abdominal wall and is used with good

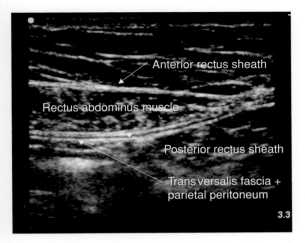

Figure 8.5.21 Cross-sectional view of anterior abdominal wall showing rectus abdominus muscle, anterior and posterior rectus sheath, transversalis fascia and parietal peritoneum.

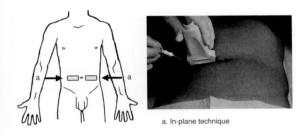

a. In-plane technique

Figure 8.5.22 Rectus sheath block, positioning and technique.

effect in children and adults following umbilical hernia surgery and is increasingly popular following laparoscopic surgery and limited upper abdominal incisions [42]. The sensory nerves for the anterior abdominal wall pierce the posterior rectus sheath and supply the skin over the medial part of the abdominal wall.

The classical technique for this has been a pop–scratch technique in which the needle is felt to "pop" as it passes through the anterior rectus sheath and "scratch" to feel the posterior rectus sheath – where local anesthetic is injected (Figure 8.5.21).

With ultrasound, the rectus abdominus muscle is easily and clearly seen. At the level of the umbilicus the posterior rectus sheath is identified and the needle inserted in an in-plane approach to the anterior surface of the posterior rectus sheath. Local anesthetic is injected to distend this space – in adults 10–20 ml of local anesthetic per side (Figure 8.5.22).

REFERENCES

1. Bombeli T, Spahn DR. Updates in perioperative coagulation: physiology and management of thromboembolism and haemorrhage. *British Journal of Anaesthesia* 2004;93:275–87.

2. Chayen D, Nathan H, Chayen M. The psoas compartment block. *Anesthesiology* 1976;45:95–9.

3. Lirk P, Kirchmair L, Prassl A *et al.* 25 years of psoas compartment block: does the psoas compartment really exist? *British Journal of Anaesthesia* 2001;87:37.

4. Berry M, Bannister LH, Standring SM. Nervous system. In: Williams PL, Bannister LH, Berry M, eds. *Grays Anatomy*. New York, Churchill Livingstone. 1995;1277–82.

5. Farny J, Drolet P, Girard M. Anatomy of the posterior approach to the lumbar plexus block. *Canadian Journal of Anaesthesia* 1994;41:480–5.

6. Hanna MH, Peat SJ, d'Costa F. Lumbar plexus block: an anatomical study. *Anaesthesia* 1993;48:675–8.

7. Winnie AP, Ramamurthy S, Durrany Z, Radonjic R. Plexus blocks for lower extremity surgery. *Anesthesia Review* 1974;1:11–6.

8. Parkinson SK, Mueller JB, Little WL, Bailey SL. Extent of blockade with various approaches to the lumbar plexus. *Anesthesia and Analgesia* 1989;68:243–8.

9. Aida S, Takahashi H, Shimoji K. Renal subcapsular hematoma after lumbar plexus block. *Anesthesiology* 1996;84:452–5.

10. Kirchmair L, Entner T, Wissel J, *et al.* A study of the paravertebral anatomy for ultrasound-guided posterior lumbar plexus block. *Anesthesia and Analgesia* 2001;93: 477–81, fourth contents page.

11. Kirchmair L, Enna B, Mitterschiffthaler G, *et al.* Lumbar plexus in children. A sonographic study and its relevance to pediatric regional anesthesia. *Anesthesiology* 2004;101:445–50.

12. Kirchmair L, Entner T, Kapral S, Mitterschiffthaler G. Ultrasound guidance for the psoas compartment block: an imaging study. *Anesthesia and Analgesia* 2002;94: 706–10; table of contents.

13. Jamieson RW, Swigart LL, Anson BJ. Points of parietal perforation of the ilioinguinal and iliohypogastric nerves in relation to optimal sites for local anaesthesia. *Quarterly Bulletin of the Northwest University Medical School* 1952; 26:22–6.

14. Niesel HC. Regionalanästhesie an Kopf und Stamm. In: Niesel HC, ed. *Regionalanästhesie, Lokalanästhesie, Regionale Schmerztherapie.* 1 ed. Stuttgart, Georg Thieme Verlag. 1994; 535–8.

15. Ang BL. Transient quadriceps paresis after ilioinguinal nerve block. *Singapore Medical Journal* 1997;38:83–4.

16. Ghani KR, McMillan R, Paterson-Brown S. Transient femoral nerve palsy following ilio-inguinal nerve blockade for day case inguinal hernia repair. *Journal of the Royal College of Surgeons Edinburgh* 2002;47:626–9.

17. Johr M, Sossai R. Colonic puncture during ilioinguinal nerve block in a child. *Anesthesia and Analgesia* 1999;88:1051–2.

18. Vaisman J. Pelvic hematoma after an ilioinguinal nerve block for orchialgia. *Anesthesia and Analgesia* 2001;92: 1048–9.

19. Lim SL, Ng Sb A, Tan GM. Ilioinguinal and iliohypogastric nerve block revisited: single shot versus double shot technique for hernia repair in children. *Paediatric Anaesthesia* 2002;12:255–60.

20. Marhofer P, Schrogendorfer K, Koinig H *et al.* Ultrasonographic guidance improves sensory block and onset time of three-in-one blocks. *Anesthesia and Analgesia* 1997;85:854–7.

21. Marhofer P, Schrogendorfer K, Wallner T, *et al.* Ultrasonographic guidance reduces the amount of local anesthetic for 3-in-1 blocks. *Regional Anesthesia and Pain Medicine* 1998;23:584–8.

22. Marhofer P, Schrogendorfer K, Andel H, *et al.* [Combined sciatic nerve-3 in 1 block in high risk patient]. *Anästhesiologie, Intensivmedizin, Notfallmedizin, Schmerztherapie* 1998;33: 399–401.

23. De Mey JC, Deruyck LJ, Cammu G, *et al.* A paravenous approach for the saphenous nerve block. *Regional Anesthesia and Pain Medicine* 2001;26:504–6.

24. Taboada M, Lorenzo D, Oliveira J, *et al.* [Comparison of 4 techniques for internal saphenous nerve block]. *Revista española de Anestesiología y reanimacíon* 2004;51:509–14.

25. Bridenbaugh PO. The lower extremity: somatic blockade. In: Cousins MJ, ed. *Neural Blockade in Clinical Anaesthesia and Management of Pain.* Philadelphia, Lippincott. 1980;320–42.

26. Stone BA. Transcutaneous stimulation of the saphenous nerve to locate injection site. *Regional Anesthesia and Pain Medicine* 2003;28:153–4.

27. Poehling GG, Bassett FH, 3rd, Goldner JL. Arthroscopy: its role in treating nontraumatic and traumatic lesions of the knee. *Southern Medical Journal* 1977;70:465–9.

28. Marhofer P, Greher M, Kapral S. Ultrasound guidance in regional anaesthesia. *British Journal of Anaesthesia* 2005;94:7–17.

29. Graif M, Seton A, Nerubai J, *et al.* Sciatic nerve: sonographic evaluation and anatomic-pathologic considerations. *Radiology* 1991;181:405–8.

30. Raj PP, Parks RI, Watson TD, Jenkins MT. A new single-position supine approach to sciatic-femoral nerve block. *Anesthesia and Analgesia* 1975;54:489–93.

31. Bergmann R, Thompson S, Afifi A, Saadeh F. *Compendium of Human Anatomy Variation.* München, Urban & Schwarzenberg. 1988;494–9.

32. Di Benedetto P, Casati A, Bertini L, Fanelli G. Posterior subgluteal approach to block the sciatic nerve: description of the technique and initial clinical experiences. *European Journal of Anaesthesiology* 2002;19:682–6.

33. Triado VD, Crespo MT, Aguilar JL, *et al.* A comparison of lateral popliteal versus lateral midfemoral sciatic nerve blockade using ropivacaine 0.5%. *Regional Anesthesia and Pain Medicine* 2004;29:23–7.

34. Pham Dang C. Midfemoral block: a new lateral approach to the sciatic nerve. *Anesthesia and Analgesia* 1999;88:1426.

35. Konrad C, Johr M. Blockade of the sciatic nerve in the popliteal fossa: a system for standardization in children. *Anesthesia and Analgesia* 1998;87:1256–8.

36. Tobias JD, Mencio GA. Popliteal fossa block for postoperative analgesia after foot surgery in infants and children. *Journal of Pediatric Orthopaedics* 1999;19:511–4.

37. Domingo Triado V, Cabezudo de la Muela L, Crespo Pociello MT, *et al.* [Sciatic nerve block with 1% mepivacaine for foot surgery: posterior versus lateral approach to the popliteal fossa]. *Revista española de Anestesiología y Reanimación* 2004;51:70–4.

38. Schwemmer U, Markus, CK, Greim CA, *et al.* Sonographic imaging of the sciatic nerve and its division in the popliteal fossa in children. *Paediatric Anaesthesia* 2004;14:1005–8.

39. Rivas Ferreira E, Sala-Blanch X, Bargallo X, *et al.* [Ultrasound-guided posterior approach to block the sciatic nerve at the popliteal fossa]. *Revista española de Anestesiología y Reanimación* 2004;51:604–7.

40. Sites BD, Gallagher J, Sparks M. Ultrasound-guided popliteal block demonstrates an atypical motor response to nerve stimulation in 2 patients with diabetes mellitus. *Regional Anesthesia and Pain Medicine* 2003;28:479–82.

41. Dabbas Nayef A, Zuzuarregui Girones JC, Arnal Bertome MC, *et al.* [Lateral popliteal block: a modification of anatomical references]. *Revista española de Anestesiología y Reanimación* 2003;50:126–9.

42. Dolan J, Lucie P, Geary T, Smith M, Kenny G. The rectus sheath block for laparoscopic surgery in adults: a comparison between the loss of resistance and the ultrasound guided techniques. *Anaesthesia* 2007;Mar:62(3): 302.

Chapter 9

Use of ultrasound to aid local anesthetic nerve blocks in children

AMY WALKER AND STEVE ROBERTS

Introduction

The use of ultrasound (US) in medicine has increased dramatically in recent years. NICE guidelines in 2002 recommended the use of US to guide placement of central venous catheters. This led to an increased availability of portable machines. Due to improved and cheaper technology, interest in its application to facilitate regional anesthesia accelerated.

The benefits of regional anesthesia are well-documented. However, "blind" blocks that rely on anatomical landmarks and/or fascial clicks (e.g. rectus sheath) can cause serious complications. Nerve-stimulating techniques may not be as safe as originally thought, as it is possible for the needle to be intraneuronal without stimulating the motor component, and subsequently not produce a twitch. The key requirement for a successful block is optimal distribution of local anesthetic (LA) around nerve structures. This goal is most effectively achieved under sonographic visualization. The development of high-resolution portable US, and the improved understanding of sonographic anatomy, have made US for regional anesthesia feasible.

Advantages of ultrasound

- No ionizing radiation.
- Identifies target nerves and important surrounding structures, e.g. pleura.

- Real-time needle guidance and observation of LA distribution.
- Faster onset of block and higher success rates.
- Allows assessment of catheter position by observing injectate or 1 ml of air.
- Blocks can be repeated if surgery is prolonged unexpectedly.
- Can be used in patients who have been given muscle relaxants.

Additional advantages in children

- Allows anatomical assessment in situations where congenital abnormalities can lead to misleading or absent surface landmarks.
- Lower volumes of LA can be used (allowing multiple blocks, and reducing the risk of LA toxicity).
- Blocks are performed under general anesthetic (GA) when the signs and symptoms of complications when awake may be masked.
- Nerves are more superficial; therefore, higher-frequency probes (10 MHz plus) can be used.
- Better neuroaxial imaging is achieved due to less ossification.

Disadvantages of ultrasound

- Loss of resolution with greater depth.
- Anisotropy (see below).
- Ossification prevents passage of US.

Ultrasound in Anesthetic Practice, ed. Graham Arthurs and Barry Nicholls. Published by Cambridge University Press.
© Cambridge University Press 2009.

- Specific training required.
- Long learning curve (block-dependent).
- Relatively expensive equipment.

What do tissues look like with ultrasound?

Substances with a high water content (e.g. blood, CSF) are very good conductors of sound and reflect very little (this is why pregnant women are asked to have a full bladder for obstetric scans). They are described as echolucent, hypoechoic, or anechoic, and appear as dark areas. Substances such as bone and air that contain little or no water reflect almost all the energy and appear very bright; they are described as hyperechoic. Tissues that conduct sound to a degree in between these extremes will appear in shades of gray depending on the amount of energy they reflect.

Arteries and veins will be anechoic and appear circular in transverse section or tubular in longitudinal section. Arteries are pulsatile and non-compressible (although small superficial arteries may sometimes seem compressible) and veins are easily compressed. You may see an area of greater echogenicity deep to the vessels in transverse section that may be mistaken for nerve tissue. This is known as post-cystic enhancement.

Nerves are collections of axons (fascicles) surrounded by connective tissue. In transverse view, they tend to be circular or oval (although they can become more triangular or flattened if they are squashed between muscles) with a bright surface (the epineurium). Internally there are multiple hypoechoic black dots (the nerve fascicles) with bright outlines (the perineurium). In a longitudinal view, the nerves are tubular structures with a bright surface and numerous discontinuous hypo- and hyperechoic lines within. One problem with identifying peripheral nerves is that they can look very dissimilar in different parts of the body. The sonographic appearance of peripheral nerves may vary significantly from nerve to nerve and even within the course of a single nerve. A second problem with identifying nerve tissue is that they display anisotropy. For a nerve image to be generated, the US beam must hit the nerve and rebound back to the probe. Nerves are very reflective (anisotropic) and may be poorly imaged or not seen at all if the probe is not placed in a perpendicular position.

Tendons have a fibrillar appearance. They generally appear more echodense/hyperechoic than nerves, and are less anisotropic. Tendons tend to be located below the level of nerves, closer to the bone, and passive or active movement of the limb may produce noticeable movement.

Pleura appear as one or two hyperechoic lines. When two are present they are seen to glide over one another with respiration.

Equipment
The ultrasound machine
Most ultrasound machines used in anesthesia are laptop-sized, cart-based machines. There are a number of features common to many machines and it is important to be familiar with these functions before you begin scanning.

- Settings – depending upon the probe selected and the capabilities of the machine you will have a number of tissue-type options. On basic machines choose a "small parts" or "superficial" setting; on more sophisticated machines, a "nerve" setting is available.
- Probe frequency – the attached probes are broadband in nature, which means they have a range of frequencies; the frequency is selected on the machine.
- Depth markers – each probe has a maximum and minimum depth. You can adjust the depth on the machine. There are 0.5 cm or 1 cm markers on the screen. These can be used to estimate the depth of structures.
- Orientation – in the left-hand corner of the screen there will be a dot or icon. This

correlates to a marker (usually a groove) on the probe. Some machines allow the dot to be positioned at the top or bottom as well as on the left or right. This is not particularly useful for nerve blocks and you should keep the dot at the top. To double check screen-probe orientation, gently tap one end of the probe to elicit a response on the screen.

- Gain – most machines allow you to adjust near and far gain as well as overall gain. This basically allows you to adjust the brightness of the image. To optimize gain, ensure vessels on screen are anechoic and that the rest of the image is of a uniform brightness. More advanced machines have "autogain" and do this for you.

- Tissue harmonics – more advanced machines exhibit this feature to improve deep image quality. Conventional ultrasound imaging sends out a fundamental beam and receives essentially the same frequency range back as an echo. Deep structures are imaged with low frequencies: these waves become distorted as the tissue expands and compresses in response. When a certain energy level is reached, this distortion results in the generation of additional frequencies, called harmonics. These higher harmonic frequencies return to the transducer together with the fundamental frequency. The second harmonic (twice the frequency of the fundamental) is used for harmonic imaging. Although the harmonic signal is weaker it better retains its purity by only having to travel one way from within the tissue to the receiver. By electronic filtering, the harmonic frequency is isolated, and can be used to create an image with enhanced contrast and gray tone differentiation.

- Multi-beam technology – provides increased contrast resolution, enhanced border visualization, decreased clutter levels and improved needle visualization. The US beam is fired in a number of planes from the transducer; if a signal is seen only in one plane, it is discounted as artifact.

- Still and video image collection – useful for training.

- Measurement tools – callipers, circumference and cross-sectional areas.

- Multidocking – for convenience, three probes can be attached at once.

- Mobile stand – for transporting the machine, storing extra probes, gel and other equipment.

Probe selection

This will depend on the structure you are looking for, as there is an inverse relationship between frequency and depth of penetration. High-frequency probes (10–14 MHz) have limited penetration (3–4 cm), but produce high-resolution images; this is excellent news for the pediatric population, as most nerves are very superficial. Low-frequency probes (3–5 MHz) can be used to image deeper structures, but will provide lower-resolution images.

US probes are described according to the arrangement of their piezo-electric elements.

- In a *linear* probe the piezo-electric crystals are arranged in a straight line, the US beams travel in parallel, creating a field that is as wide as the probe length (footprint). They are suitable for most nerve blocks.

- A *curvilinear* array has a curved surface, creating a field in depth that is wider than the footprint of the probe, making it possible to create a smaller footprint for easier access through small windows. This results in a wider field at depth, but reduces lateral resolution as the scan lines diverge. It is of particular use for deep blocks, e.g. the gluteal approach to the sciatic nerve.

The size of the footprint (or probe length) needs to be suitable for the size of the patient and the type of block you are performing. For example, a hockey-stick probe (25 mm length) will be best for an ilioinguinal block in a baby, but you may choose a 38 mm length probe for the same baby if you want to thread a caudal catheter, as it will allow a greater field of vision.

Needle selection

Short bevelled needles are preferable. They give the operator a better sense of feel through tissue, and a more convincing "pop" as the needle passes through fascial layers. In addition, the injection port is at the tip of the needle allowing more accurate deposit of LA. The shape of the needle tip makes intraneural positioning more difficult, although if this does occur it may cause greater damage. Most makes of needle image equally well, although larger needles will reflect more. It is important to remember that the more parallel the needle is to the probe, the more visible it will be.

Basic principles

- Check the weight of the patient and consider the appropriate dose of LA (see below).
- Obtain consent from the patient/parents. Give an explanation of the potential advantages, side effects, complications and methods of pain relief if the block fails.
- Consider giving paracetamol and a non-steroidal anti-inflammatory drug (NSAID) pre-operatively.
- Occasionally children are operated on awake. The presence of a parent or play specialist may be useful: they can be distracted with audiovisual aids, e.g. MP3 player. Ametop can be applied to the proposed puncture site pre-operatively. Entonox may be used during block insertion.
- As with all blocks, IV access, appropriate monitoring, resuscitation facilities, aseptic technique, and the presence of a trained assistant are essential.
- Take time to position the patient, the machine and yourself so that you can see the screen comfortably.
- Choose the appropriate probe based on depth of target nerve and size of patient.

- Set the machine for "small parts" or "nerve", and the highest resolution possible for the target depth.
- Set the depth greater than you expect to find the nerve of interest to avoid missing it.
- Orientate the probe with the screen and the patient (in other words, make sure what you think is medial actually *is* medial).
- Dim the lights.
- Use lots of ultrasound gel.
- Get used to scanning with your non-dominant hand. You will need your dominant hand for needling.
- Your scanning hand should rest on the patient – this prevents the probe, and therefore the image, from drifting.
- Try to develop a survey pattern for each nerve using landmarks and borders that you can follow every time.
- Keep the target in the middle depth of the screen. This will make it easier to introduce the needle in an appropriate position.

Infection precautions

For *single puncture* a surface disinfectant (compatible with the manufacturer's recommendations) is used on the transducer. The patient's skin is cleaned in the usual manner and sterile ultrasound gel is applied. A no-touch strategy is employed. An alternative is to place a sterile dressing (excluding all air bubbles) over the probe.

For *perineural catheter insertion* a full aseptic technique is used, with the operator gloved and gowned, sterile drapes and a sterile sheath for the ultrasound probe. Ultrasound gel is applied twice, once inside the sheath and again outside.

Needling technique

There are two options for introducing the needle:
- An in-plane approach (IP) – also called in-line or long axis. The needle is introduced along the long axis of the probe. The whole needle is visualized

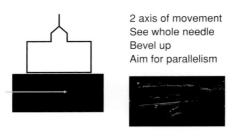

2 axis of movement
See whole needle
Bevel up
Aim for parallelism

Figure 9.1   Needle in-plane.

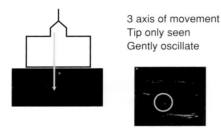

3 axis of movement
Tip only seen
Gently oscillate

Figure 9.2   Needle out-of-plane.

providing the needle and US beam are kept in perfect alignment (Figure 9.1).

- An out-of-plane approach (OOP) – also called cross-sectional, short axis or transverse approach. The needle is introduced across the short axis of the probe as for vascular access. The tip may be seen as a hyperechoic dot; usually tip position is gauged by observing tissue movement (Figure 9.2).
- We do not recommend "blunting" a hypodermic needle, which seems to be popular in some institutions.
- It is often useful to make a small nick in the skin with a sharp needle before introducing the short bevelled needle. This will help you to avoid missing any fascial layers.
- A short bevelled needle with flexible injection tubing is suitable for most peripheral nerve block techniques.
- Remove all the air from the injectate and needle (air will absorb 99% of US).
- Introduce the needle bevel up.
- If unsure, use PNS to confirm nerve and needle position. Set the PNS for 0.5 mA or 1.0 mA

and do not adjust the current during the block.

- Aspirate, then inject 0.5–1 ml of LA; if fascial plane around nerve begins to open up then inject more LA; continue to observe spread. It should spread circumferentially about the nerve.
- The injection should be done slowly with frequent aspiration to exclude intravascular injection.
- With an OOP technique perform injections at 3 and 9 o'clock.
- With an IP approach perform injections at 6 *and then at* 12 o'clock.
- When using the IP technique, it may be prudent to move your intended target so it is positioned in the third of the screen furthest from your needle entry point. This way the needle does not appear suddenly on the screen by the nerve.
- With the IP technique, the needle should enter the skin at a depth equal to the depth of the nerve on the US screen, this way the needle will be parallel.
- Never insert the needle if you are unsure of its position; if you lose the needle check your hands first.
- Catheters should be threaded 3 cm beyond the needle tip.
- Catheters are at risk of displacement and should be tunnelled. Remove the needle from an appropriately sized cannula. Insert the needle through the exit point of the catheter and bring it out a few centimeters lateral in a suitable position (think about how the patient will be positioned for surgery and how they will be lying postoperatively). Thread the cannula back over the needle tip, and then remove the needle. Finally thread the catheter through the cannula before removing it.

Local anesthetic doses

Neonates and small infants are prone to local anesthetic toxicity because of an immature blood–brain

Table 9.1 Doses of local anesthetic

Drug	Single-shot (mg/kg)	Continuous infusion (mg/(kg h))	Maximum dose per 4 h period (mg/kg)
Levobupivicaine	2	0.125–0.375	2.0
Ropivicaine	2	0.4	1.6
Lignocaine	3	NA	NA

barrier, decreased protein binding, and immature liver metabolic systems. It has been suggested that the dose of LA should be halved in this group (Table 9.1). Toxicity relates to the rate of rise in plasma concentration as well as the absolute dose of LA. The safest option remains levobupivicaine, which combines a long duration of action with a low risk of cardio- and neurotoxicity.

Contraindications
Absolute
- Lack of consent.
- Allergy to LA.
- Infection at the site of needle introduction.

Relative
- Systemic infection (catheter techniques).
- Bleeding disorders (US may decrease risk).
- Neuromuscular disorders.
- Risk of compartment syndrome, particularly after trauma (discuss with surgeon).

Post-operative care
Both the patient and the parents must be warned pre-operatively that the child may experience numbness, weakness and heaviness of a blocked limb. It is particularly important to warn parents that the child will not feel temperature sensation in the usual way. Ideally a blocked arm should be kept in a sling. Provision should be made for children with lower limb blocks to mobilize and return home when appropriate. Both written and verbal instructions should be issued prior to discharge, along with a warning that if the block lasts longer than 24 h they should contact the hospital. There should be a contact telephone number available at all times for parents to call with questions or concerns.

Children with continuous infusions running should be treated in a similar way to patients with an epidural – regular observations and site checks. A pain team should review them daily. Neonates and infants should have infusions discontinued after 48 h because of the risk of LA toxicity.

Training tips
- There are two skills to learn – scanning and needle–probe coordination.
- Scanning: practice on yourself and anyone else you can get to volunteer. Use your forearm to learn.
- Needle probe manipulation: this can be practiced using a vascular US phantom; pretend the "vessel" is a nerve; practise both OOP an IP approaches.
- Go on a course.
- Utilize internet resources: www.nysora.com and www.neuraxiom.com are excellent.
- Only move onto patients when you have mastered these skills.
- Start with simple blocks, e.g. femoral, and begin with teenagers.

Specific blocks
Brachial plexus blocks
Numerous techniques for blocking the brachial plexus have been described. Here we will concentrate on just two, the axillary and the supraclavicular approach.

Axillary brachial plexus block

This is an ideal block for beginners. Although it is a difficult area to scan because of the complexity of the anatomy, it is a common block and has a low complication rate. It is essential that you follow a scanning routine so that you are not initially overwhelmed.

Indications

Forearm and hand surgery.

Anatomy

The brachial plexus is formed by the anterior portions of the C5–T1 nerve roots. The roots pass through the intervertebral foramina and begin their descent towards the first rib. The trunks of the brachial plexus pass between the anterior and middle scalene muscles. They converge to form three (superior, medial and inferior) trunks, which bifurcate into anterior and posterior divisions at the supraclavicular level. Having crossed the first rib, they separate into posterior, lateral and median cords before forming the terminal nerves.

Sonoanatomy

In the axilla and the upper arm, the neurovascular bundle is located in the internal bicipital sulcus, which separates the flexor muscle compartment (biceps and coracobrachialis muscles) from the extensor compartment (triceps). The most easily identified structure is the round pulsatile axillary artery. Up to five veins can be found in the axilla. The location of nerves in the axilla can be variable. The nerves are round to oval shaped, and hypoechoic with internal hyperechoic areas. The median and ulnar nerves are usually lateral and medial to the artery, respectively. The radial nerve is often posterior or postero-medial to the artery. The musculocutaneous nerve usually branches off more proximally, and can be seen as a hyperechoic ellipse between the biceps and coracobrachialis muscles

TIPS:
1. OOP or IP
2. Ballot
3. If in doubt, inject perivascular and find musculocutaneous
4. Beware post-cystic enhancement

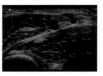

NB radial nerve not visible on these US images

Figure 9.3 Axillary approach.

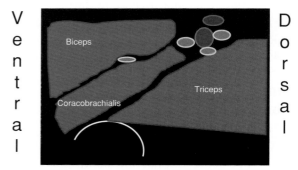

Figure 9.4 Schematic diagram of the position of the brachial plexus in the axilla.

for a short distance before entering the body of the coracobrachialis muscle (Figure 9.3).

Performance (see Figures 9.4–9.7 and video 9.8; Figures 9.5, 9.7 and video 9.8 are on the DVD)

- Position yourself, the patient and the screen ergonomically.
- Position the patient supine with his/her arm abducted to 90° and the elbow flexed.
- It is usual for the operator to stand at the head of the patient on the side of the operation.
- Place the screen by the patient's chest on the operative side.
- First, identify the humerus.
- Then find the axillary artery and vein (confirm with color-flow Doppler).
- Compress the veins.

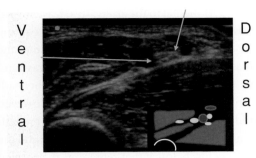

Figure 9.6 Ultrasound image of the position of the brachial plexus in the axilla. Arrows are lines of the needles.

- Next find the musculocutaneous nerve. It is usually very easy to see as a hyperechoic ellipse between the biceps and coracobrachialis muscles. As you move the probe into the axilla, the nerve travels inwards towards the artery; as the probe is moved distal the ellipse travels away from the artery and its shape becomes triangular.
- Now look more closely around the artery.
- Remember to change the angle of the probe; imagine the course of the nerve and position your probe in a perpendicular position to the nerves course: they will not be traveling parallel to the skin. The nerves are anisotropic.
- The median nerve should be lateral to the artery (closest to the musculocutaneous nerve); the ulna is usually the most medial structure, and the radial may be found in the posterior or postero-lateral position.
- Don't mistake the hyperechoic shadow beneath the artery for a nerve – it may be post-cystic enhancement.
- Ballot the skin; in doing so, the nerves can sometimes be seen to move around the artery.
- Following the structures down the arm may help you identify the nerves. The median nerve should remain close to the artery and often swaps sides; the ulnar nerve is very superficial and moves away from the artery.

- The radial nerve passes posteriorly where it runs in the spiral groove of the humerus (Figure 9.9, on DVD).
- Either an OOP or an IP technique can be used.
- Block the deepest nerves first to avoid distortion of the more superficial structures (usually radial, ulna, median then musculocutaneous).
- You may find that the nerves become more obvious as the LA is injected.
- In small children, the musculocutaneous nerve will be very close to the median nerve and the LA injected to block the median nerve may be sufficient to surround it (Figure 9.10, on DVD).
- 0.1–0.3 ml/kg of LA is usually sufficient for an axillary brachial plexus block.
- If you are struggling ensure the artery is surrounded by LA, then place a few milliliters of LA on the musculocutaneous.

Potential complications
Arterial puncture, nerve damage.

Supraclavicular brachial plexus block
This is for experienced US operators only
Despite its reputation for rapid onset and dense, predictable anesthesia, this block is not commonly performed. This is because of the risk of serious complications such as pneumothorax and subclavian artery puncture. The advent of US allows the operator to see both the plexus *and* the structures to avoid, thus improving safety. A block at this level may avoid the inevitable phrenic nerve block seen with an interscalene approach.

Indications
Surgery on the upper extremity not involving the shoulder

Sonoanatomy (see Figures 9.11–9.15 and video 9.16; Figures 9.13, 9.15 and video 9.16 are on the DVD)
The subclavian artery is round and pulsatile and lies directly on the first rib. The subclavian vein is

TIPS

1. Experts only
2. IP
3. Keep artery and pleura in view
4. If difficult scan proximally into interscalene region
5. Look for dorsal scapular artery

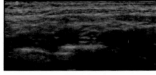

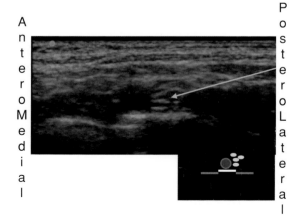

Figure 9.11 Supraclavicular block.

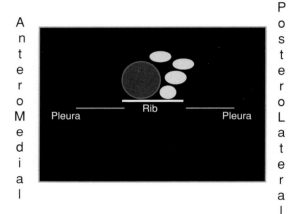

Figure 9.12 Schematic diagram of the supraclavicular position of the brachial plexus.

Figure 9.14 Ultrasound image of the supraclavicular position of the brachial plexus with needle position. Arrow is line of needle.

found antero-medial to the artery. In at least 50% of patients, the dorsal scapular artery is seen coming off the subclavian artery and passing through the brachial plexus. Usually, bone reflects ultrasound energy so completely that anything lying beneath it in an ultrasound picture is obscured. However, in children the cortical layer of ribs is thin enough that you can see both layers of the rib cortex and the bright layer just below it that represents the parietal and visceral pleura interface. The sliding sign of the pleura should be observed (Figure 9.16, on DVD).

Performance

- Position yourself, the patient and the screen ergonomically.
- The patient should be semi-sitting (this reduces the venous pressure in the neck), with the head turned slightly away from the side you intend to block.
- Use a high-frequency linear probe: a hockey stick probe is usually suitable due to its small footprint.
- Place the probe behind the clavicle looking down into the chest.
- The subclavian artery will be antero-medial. Look for the subclavian vein medial to this, and use color Doppler to confirm. Scan medial to lateral and back again, looking for the dorsal scapular artery.
- Immediately behind and above the artery sit four or more round hypoechoic circles ("bunch of grapes") – the brachial plexus.
- They can be followed proximally into the interscalene space. The nerve roots align vertically as they travel between the scalene muscles.
- When the plexus is difficult to identify, it can be useful to find the nerve roots higher in the neck and follow them down.
- Before you begin the block you must have identified the subclavian artery and the lung; *both* these structures should be kept in view.

- An IP technique is ideal as it allows greater needle control.
- Introduce the needle from the postero-lateral aspect of the probe directing it antero-medially.
- Position the needle within the sheath. It may sometimes be necessary to reposition the needle to ensure good spread.
- If this block is being used for hand surgery, it is important to get the inferior trunk, which is situated in the most dangerous area in the angle between the artery and rib/pleura.
- Doses of LA as low as 0.1–0.2 ml/kg can be used successfully.

Potential complications
- Pneumothorax (up to 6.1% for "blind" techniques).
- Phrenic nerve block (∼50%).
- Horner's syndrome.
- Intravascular injection with LA toxicity.
- Neurological injury (rare).

Lower limb blocks
The nerves of the lower limb are more difficult to scan.

Femoral nerve block
Indications
Anterior thigh and knee surgery

Anatomy
The femoral nerve arises from the L2–4 and is the largest branch of the lumbar plexus. It runs in the groove between the psoas major and iliacus muscles, with a covering of these muscles' fascia. The femoral nerve is often oval or triangular in shape and as it passes underneath the inguinal ligament it lies immediately lateral to the femoral artery. Because the nerve has two fascial layers covering it below the inguinal ligament (fascia lata and fascia iliaca), compared to the femoral artery, which is only covered by one (fascia lata), the nerve will lie

TIPS:
1. OOP
2. Probe parallel to inguinal ligament
3. Nerve often not visible
4. Inject below fascia iliaca

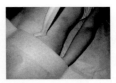
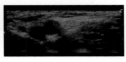

Figure 9.17 Femoral nerve block.

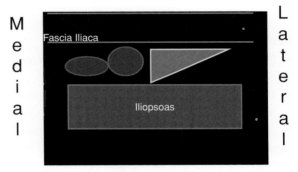

Figure 9.18 Schematic diagram of the position of the femoral nerve.

in a different tissue plane to the artery. This may explain the high failure rate of a "blind perivascular" injection.

Sonoanatomy (see Figures 9.17–9.21 and video 9.22; Figures 9.19, 9.21 and video 9.22 are on the DVD)
The femoral vessels are easily identified; the artery is pulsatile and non-compressible, with the compressible vein lying medially. Scanning distally reveals branches of these vessels. The nerve is a variable distance lateral to the artery; it appears oval, although occasionally it is triangular. The nerve itself is often not distinct as it is surrounded by fat; the fat and nerve create a *triangle* with its base adjacent to the artery (Figure 9.19, on DVD).

M
e
d
i
a
l

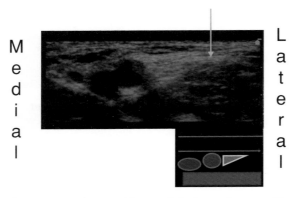

L
a
t
e
r
a
l

Figure 9.20 Ultrasound image of the femoral nerve with needle position. Arrow is line of needle.

Performance

- Position yourself, the patient and the screen ergonomically.
- The patient should be supine. In infants it may help to place a small roll under the hip.
- Use a high-frequency linear probe; a hockey stick probe is appropriate for infants.
- Place the probe parallel to and on the inguinal ligament. The nerve is least likely to have divided into its branches at this point and will be easiest to see.
- First identify the vessels. The femoral artery is round, pulsatile (use color-flow Doppler) and usually smaller than the vein which lies below and medial to it.
- If the probe is too low you may see a second artery (profunda femoris) below the superficial one. Move the probe cephalad and the vessels will merge.
- An OOP technique should be used.
- Aim your needle at the lateral point of the triangle. This keeps the vessels at a safe distance and means you are not aiming directly at the nerve structures.
- For success, the LA must be deposited beneath the fascia iliaca. The fascia is a complex structure rather like filo pastry; hence more than one "pop" may be felt. A "pop" is felt as you enter

the fascia iliaca, aspirate then inject a milliliter of LA and observe the spread. If the LA does not spread medially towards the artery then the needle needs to be advanced a fraction further. Another "pop" will be felt and the process is repeated until optimal spread occurs.

- 0.1–0.2 ml/kg of LA is adequate.

Potential complications

Vascular injection, hematoma, and nerve injury.

Sciatic nerve block

The sciatic nerve may be blocked at any point along its course, but the two most popular approaches are subgluteal and popliteal.

Popliteal approach

Indications

Ankle and foot surgery (may require saphenous nerve block).

Anatomy

The popliteal fossa is a diamond-shaped space at the posterior aspect of the knee. The biceps femoris muscle forms its supero-lateral border and the semitendinosus and semimembranosus muscles its supero-medial border. The two heads of the gastrocnemius muscle form the inferior borders.

The tibial nerve (the larger of the two divisions of the sciatic nerve) emerges at the upper apex of the popliteal fossa, between the diverging hamstrings, and runs straight down to its lower apex. It lies superficial and lateral to the deeper popliteal vein and artery (deeper than the vein). The common peroneal nerve lies more superficial and lateral still to the tibial nerve. It runs medial to the biceps femoris muscle before moving anteriorly into the peroneus longus muscle where it lies against the neck of the fibula.

TIPS:

1. OOP or IP
2. Look superficial and lateral to vein
3. Tibial nerve is on the vein – track back
4. See-saw

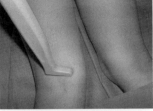

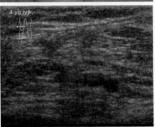

Figure 9.23 Popliteal approach to sciatic nerve.

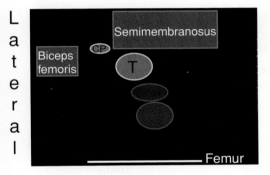

Figure 9.24 Schematic diagram of the position of the sciatic nerve in the popliteal fossa.

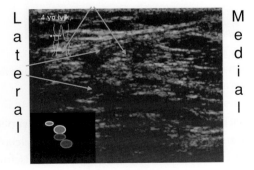

Figure 9.26 Ultrasound image of the sciatic nerve in the popliteal fossa with needle position. Arrows are lines of the needles.

Sonoanatomy (see Figures 9.23–9.27 and video 9.28; Figures 9.25, 9.27 and video 9.28 are on the DVD)

The tibial nerve lies on the popliteal vein, which lies superficial to the popliteal artery (the vessels may be difficult to see in this area so color-flow Doppler is useful). The tibial nerve is round with a typical fascicular pattern and is a similar size to the artery; the common peroneal nerve is more superficial and lateral to it. The common peroneal nerve is smaller and more hypoechoic.

Performance

- Position yourself, the patient and the screen ergonomically.
- Position the patient on their side with the leg to be blocked uppermost.
- Get everything ready before you start – the sciatic nerve can be elusive and it can be very frustrating to get a beautiful picture and be unable to produce it a second time because you had not prepared your equipment.
- A high-frequency linear probe will be suitable in all but the largest of patients (when you may need to change the setting to a lower frequency by changing from "resolution" to "general").
- Start at the popliteal crease.
- Identify the popliteal artery and vein (use Doppler, and compress).
- The sciatic nerve and its branches exhibit a high degree of anisotropy so even very small changes in the angulation of the beam will dissolve the picture.
- Focus your attention on the expected position of the tibial nerve (above and slightly lateral to the vein) and try angling your probe slightly caudad then slightly cephalad.
- More superficial and lateral still will be the common peroneal component of the sciatic nerve.
- Don't worry if you cannot see the common peroneal nerve. Trace the tibial nerve up the leg and

you should see the common peroneal move in towards it.

- It is often helpful to get an assistant to dorsiflex and plantarflex the patient's foot (see-saw sign). This stretches the two nerves alternately, and may make them easier to spot.
- Once you have identified the two nerves and the point of division, you can pick the optimal place to deposit the LA. Generally this is at a level just proximal to the division.
- Either an OOP or IP technique can be employed.
- Remember that the saphenous nerve innervates the medial aspect of the lower leg.

Potential complications

- Damage to popliteal vessels.
- Nerve damage.

Subgluteal approach
Indications
Surgery on the knee, tibia, fibula, ankle, and foot.

Anatomy
The sciatic nerve is the largest nerve in the body, measuring 2 cm in breadth in some adults. It supplies nearly the whole of the skin of the leg, the muscles of the back of the thigh, and those of the lower leg and foot. It passes from the pelvis through the greater sciatic foramen, below the piriformis muscle and along the back of the thigh to about its lower third, where it divides into two large branches, the tibial and common peroneal nerves. This division may take place at any point between the sacral plexus and the lower third of the thigh.

Sonoanatomy (see Figures 9.29–9.33 and video 9.34; Figures 9.31, 9.33 and video 9.34 are on the DVD)
The sciatic nerve is found subgluteally slightly superficial and medial to the shaft of the femur

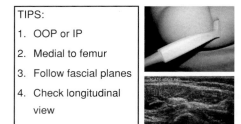

TIPS:
1. OOP or IP
2. Medial to femur
3. Follow fascial planes
4. Check longitudinal view

Figure 9.29 Subgluteal approach to the sciatic nerve.

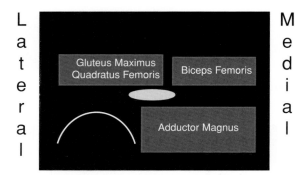

Figure 9.30 Schematic diagram of the subgluteal approach to the sciatic nerve.

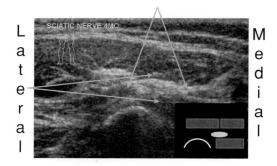

Figure 9.32 Ultrasound image of the subgluteal approach to the sciatic nerve with needle position. Arrows are lines of needle.

sandwiched between the gluteus maximus (superficial) and the quadratus femoris muscles (deep). More proximally, the bony landmarks are the ischial tuberosity (medial) and the greater trochanter (lateral). The nerve has a flattened appearance and is the most difficult nerve to identify because of its extreme anisotropic behavior. Often the posterior cutaneous nerve of the thigh can be seen medial and slightly more superficial to the sciatic nerve (Figure 9.31, on DVD).

Performance
- Position yourself, the patient and the screen ergonomically.
- Position the patient on their side with the leg to be blocked uppermost.
- It is appropriate to use a high-frequency linear probe for most blocks in children because the structures are superficial compared with adults. In a large teenager, you may need to use a lower frequency (7 MHz).
- Get everything ready before you start – the sciatic nerve shows a high degree of anisotropy and you need to be in a position to begin the block when you get a good picture.
- Place the probe transversally beneath the gluteal crease. Occasionally the nerve will be immediately obvious to you, but more often than not it will be difficult to see.
- Look for the femoral shaft and concentrate on the area medial and slightly more superficial. Follow the fascial planes into this area; the nerve is sandwiched between the muscles.
- Try angling your probe caudad and cephalad.
- If you are having difficulties, reposition the probe in a longitudinal plane. Scan lateral to medial and you should see a bright white band of tissue – the sciatic nerve. Keeping your target in the center of the screen, pivot the probe 90° to give a transverse view again. The nerve should now be visible.
- Remember when you pivot the probe to make sure that the lateral part of the probe still equates with the lateral part of the screen.
- The posterior cutaneous femoral nerve can be visualized medial and slightly more superficial to the sciatic nerve. It should be blocked if a tourniquet is to be used.

- Either an OOP or IP approach may be used; however, it is important to use a long enough needle for the latter technique.

Potential complications
Nerve damage.

Truncal blocks
Rectus sheath block
Indications
Anterior abdominal wall surgery, e.g. umbilical hernia repair.

Anatomy
The aponeuroses of the external oblique, internal oblique and transverse abdominis form the rectus sheath that encloses the rectus abdominis muscles. There are three fibrous intertendinous intersections. These are attached anteriorly to the sheath but not posteriorly. For LA to spread caudad and cephalad, the needle must be positioned just anterior to the posterior sheath. Below the arcuate line the rectus sheath is deficient posteriorly. There is very little correlation between the depth of the posterior rectus sheath with age, weight, height or surface area.

Sonoanatomy (see Figures 9.35–9.38 and video 9.39; Figure 9.38 and video 9.39 are on the DVD)
The three muscles – external oblique, internal oblique and transverse abdominis – can be easily identified laterally. More medially, the muscle layers start to thin and become aponeuroses. The point at which they join is called the semilunaris. Medial to the semilunaris, the aponeuroses split, with some fibers passing anterior to the rectus muscle and some posterior. In the midline, the aponeuroses from both sides join to form the linea alba. There will be two hyperechoic lines posterior to the rectus muscle. The more superficial one is the

141

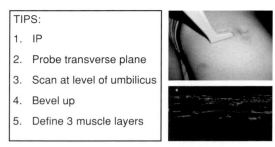

TIPS:
1. IP
2. Probe transverse plane
3. Scan at level of umbilicus
4. Bevel up
5. Define 3 muscle layers

Figure 9.35 Rectus sheath block.

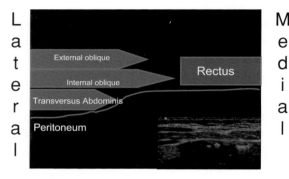

Figure 9.36 Schematic diagram of the rectus sheath block.

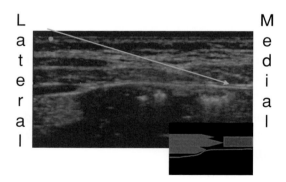

Figure 9.37 Ultrasound image of the rectus sheath block with needle position. Arrow is line of needle.

posterior part of the rectus sheath and the deeper one is the peritoneum (Figure 9.37).

Performance

- Position yourself, the patient and the screen ergonomically.
- A high-frequency linear probe is suitable.

- Place the probe in the transverse plane at the level of the umbilicus.
- Starting laterally, scan towards the midline, identifying the three muscle layers of the abdominal wall. Note the peritoneum deep to the transversus abdominis. As you scan medially, the muscle layers become aponeuroses and form the semilunaris (lateral border of the rectus sheath).
- At the semilunaris the aponeuroses split to encompass the rectus muscle.
- The linea alba lies in the midline between the two rectus muscles.
- There are two hyperechoic lines (train track) posterior to the rectus muscle. These are the posterior rectus sheath (anterior) and the peritoneum (posterior).
- This block lends itself to an IP technique.
- The needle is advanced from lateral to medial.
- The tip of the needle is positioned between the rectus muscle and its posterior fascia. Often a small give is felt as you come out of the muscle into the potential posterior space.
- The needle is positioned correctly if the rectus sheath peels away from the muscle during injection.
- In smaller children it is possible to hold the probe in the midline and block both sides without adjusting the probe.

Potential complications

Intraperitoneal injection and visceral damage.

Ilioinguinal/iliohypogastric block

Despite its popularity, no consensus has been reached on how to perform this block (one or two fascial "clicks"?), and the failure rate can be up to 30%. In addition, serious complications (e.g. intestinal puncture and pelvic hematoma) have been reported. The effectiveness of ilioinguinal/iliohypogastric nerve blockade can be greatly

TIPS

1. OOP or IP
2. Keep ASIS on screen
3. Define 3 muscle layers
4. If you can't identify the nerves, place LA in fascial plane between IO and TA

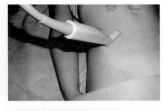

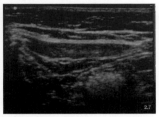

Figure 9.40 Ilioinguinal nerve block.

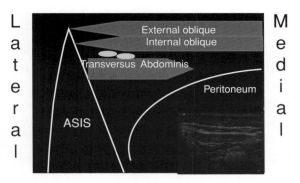

Figure 9.41 Schematic diagram of anterior abdominal wall and ilioinguinal nerve.

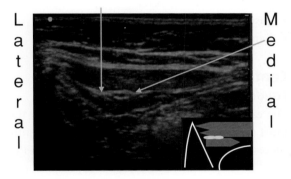

Figure 9.43 Ultrasound image of anterior abdominal wall and ilioinguinal nerve with needles in place. Arrows are lines of the needles.

improved when performed with US, despite using significantly lower amounts of LA.

Anatomy

The ilioinguinal (L1) and iliohypogastric (T12, L1) nerves are terminal branches of the lumbar plexus. They lie deep to the internal oblique. The iliohypogastric nerve pierces the internal oblique and runs under the external oblique superior to the inguinal canal. The ilioinguinal nerve continues in the inguinal canal. In infants the average nerve-peritoneum distance is only 3.3 mm.

Sonoanatomy (Figures 9.40–9.43 and video 9.44; Figure 9.42 and video 9.44 are on the DVD)

The anterior superior iliac spine (ASIS) is the most easily recognizable landmark for this block. It appears as an echolucent shadow beneath a hyperechoic peak, and should be kept at the lateral part of the screen to aid orientation. It is usually quite easy to see all three muscle layers. The nerve lies between the transversus abdominis and internal oblique muscles. The peritoneum is a bright line beneath the transversus abdominis. You may see bowel contents move with peristalsis (Figure 9.44, on DVD).

Indications

Inguinal surgery (e.g. hernia repair, orchidopexy).

Performance

- Position yourself, the patient and the machine ergonomically.
- A hockey stick probe is useful for infants.
- Place the probe on the ASIS and try to keep this landmark in view at all times (the nerve is a mean distance of only 7 mm from the ASIS in children).
- Start laterally and identify the three muscle layers.
- As you move the probe more medially, the external oblique will become aponeurosis.

- The nerve will be between the internal oblique and the transversus muscles.
- Either an IP technique (directing the needle laterally towards the ASIS) or an OOP approach can be used.
- In expert hands, it is possible to produce a successful block with as little as 0.075 ml/kg LA.
- If you have any concerns regarding the proximity of your injection to the nerve, use a higher volume of LA.

Potential complications

- Visceral perforation.
- Femoral nerve blockade (11%).

Central blocks
Caudal

The caudal anesthesia continues to be one of the most popular pediatric blocks. Despite apparently successful injection, failure of analgesia occurs in 2.8–11% of patients. The overall complication rate is reported at 1.5 : 1000. Although extremely rare, intravascular injection is a potentially disastrous complication. Correct cannula placement has been assessed by numerous techniques (the "whoosh" and "swoosh" tests, nerve stimulation, and addition of adrenaline to the injectate), none of which has become standard practice. The reliability of US assessment is limited by age (best in patients under 2 years of age).

Indications

- Lower abdominal surgery.
- Lower limb surgery.

Anatomy

The caudal epidural space is the lowest portion of the epidural system and is entered through the sacral hiatus. The sacral hiatus is a gap in the lower part of the posterior wall of the sacrum formed

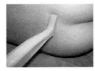
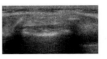

TIPS:
1. IP for fully guided
2. Locate dural sac first
3. When tracking LA injection, may need to change to paravertebral sagittal probe position

Figure 9.45 Caudal block.

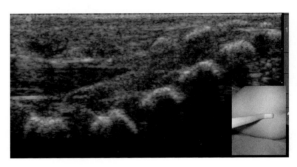

Figure 9.47 Ultrasound image of sacral canal.

by the failure of the laminae of S5 and/or S4 to fuse in the midline. The sacral canal is a continuation of the lumbar spinal canal, which terminates at the sacral hiatus. The dural sac terminates at L2 (T10–L3) in term infants, and in preterm infants at L4.

Sonoanatomy (Figures 9.45–9.49 and video 9.50; Figures 9.46, 9.49 and video 9.50 are on the DVD)

US cannot pass through bone; therefore, the neuroaxial structures can only be imaged between the bones: echo windows. Ossification increases with age, thus limiting the echo window. As you scan cephalad, these windows diminish in size. In infants, a midline sagittal probe position is adequate, with age and lumbar/thoracic scanning a paramedian position increases echo window size. The CSF is hypoechoic. The dura will be

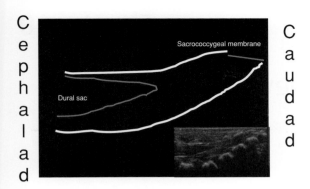

Figure 9.48 Schematic diagram of sacral canal.

hyperechoic and often appears as a double line. The cord is hypoechoic with hyperechoic walls and a hyperechoic central canal. The cauda equina is seen as numerous hyperechoic lines coming off the conus medullaris (Figure 9.47).

Performance

- Stand at the patient's back with the machine on the opposite side.
- Place the US probe in the midline sagittal position, a large footprint allows more spinal levels to be observed at a time.
- Usually US is used to assess cannula position; if placing the cannula proves difficult, then a full US-guided IP technique is advised.

- Perform a mapping scan to assess the level of the dural sac and its distance from the sacrococcygeal membrane.
- Insert the cannula perpendicular to the skin at apex of sacral hiatus; when it hits bone, re-angle to approximately 30° and insert the cannula 5 mm before sliding it off the needle.
- If the needle and the US beam are exactly aligned, it may be possible to observe the cannula.
- Aspirate, then inject 0.1–0.3 ml/kg saline (avoids wasting LA) as a test bolus. Positive placement causes the posterior dura to be displaced anteriorly.
- Then inject the LA, remembering to aspirate regularly; spread is monitored by synchronously scanning cephalad.
- US is useful for screening patients with cutaneous markers of dysraphism, allowing the anatomy to be assessed regarding suitability for caudal anesthesia.
- The main disadvantage of this technique is that as children become older ossification increases and the view of the dura becomes obscured.

Complications

- Intravascular injection.
- Spinal injection.
- Failure or inadequate block.

Chapter 10

Cranial ultrasound in the newborn

OWEN ARTHURS

Introduction

Ultrasound is now widely used to diagnose intracranial pathology in the neonate, particularly when born prematurely. Ease of access through the open fontanelles allows access to intracranial pathology with sound waves, rather than having to rely on alternative complex techniques such as computer tomography (CT) or magnetic resonance imaging (MRI). This makes it a useful and versatile ward-based tool in this particular cohort of patients, largely because of the particular pathology in this age group, typically intraventricular hemorrhages. It is safe, portable, quick and easy to perform with some basic guidance, and despite inter-user variability, even limited experience will rapidly demonstrate gross pathological changes, and so its use has also grown as a useful screening tool. This chapter concentrates on the versatility of transcranial ultrasound scanning in the newborn period.

Basic scanning principles

There are a number of basic principles that should be followed whilst undertaking transcranial ultrasound.

(1) Set the machine up correctly before you start identifying features. This includes the correct power output, receiver gain, depth gain, contrast, and zoom.

(2) The timing, and duration, of scanning in a critically unwell neonate is of great importance. It may be more important to return to the patient at a later, more stable time, than to pursue an unsatisfactory scan. Cranial ultrasound should be regarded as a life-threatening procedure in unstable infants!

(3) The entire cortex should be scanned in two dimensions: from anterior to posterior, and from left to right, reaching the skull at the extent of all sweeps.

(4) Every lesion should be definable in both planes, as it is easy to be confused by artifacts that can only be seen on one plane.

(5) Echogenic areas and interfaces appear brighter (bone, blood, ischemic areas, and calcification), whereas echolucent areas appear darker (including CSF and fluid-filled cysts).

(6) Always create a recording of the scan using video, DVD, or other format. Reviewing a tape can help revise a diagnosis, and may avoid the need to re-scan. It is much easier to review recorded moving images than static images, and these are also useful for audit and teaching purposes.

(7) Serial scans may be more useful in diagnosis than a single scan. Diagnosis is made much easier by the evolution of pathology, and daily

Ultrasound in Anesthetic Practice, ed. Graham Arthurs and Barry Nicholls. Published by Cambridge University Press.
© Cambridge University Press 2009.

scans may be required to define pathology accurately.

Basic scanning properties

Most transducers now use a 3–10 MHz probe for conventional two-dimensional real-time imaging, although the precise frequency available varies with different systems. Modern scanners use a phased linear array of quartz crystals to generate and record signals. Low frequencies (3–5 MHz) penetrate further and so are more useful for imaging deeper structures such as the posterior fossa, although resolution will be reduced. Higher frequencies (7.5–10 MHz) provide better resolution and detail at a limited depth, emphasizing cortical structures, and may be required for smaller babies.

Instrumental setup

Power output

Many scanners default to maximal power output, but the norm should be to use the minimum power output required to produce good images. Most modern ultrasound machines produce negligible power for conventional scanning (much more during Doppler scanning) and therefore maximal power may be used, but may not be entirely necessary.

Receiver gain

The receiver gains are frequently used incorrectly. There are two controls that affect the overall appearance of the image. The overall gain makes the whole image appear too dark or too light if set too low or too high, respectively. The differential depth gain is used to control the contrast at different depths in the image.

Contrast

The overall contrast can be set independently of the gain. Whereas during echocardiography a relatively high gain is required, during cranial ultrasound for parenchymal lesions, a relatively low contrast overall is required for good gray-scale differentiation.

Zoom and focus

These are two functions used to magnify the image so that it fills the entire screen: the zoom function magnifies the image, and the focus narrows the field of view, to maximize image clarity.

Other functions

Other functions such as printing, recording and taking measurements will vary according to manufacturer but are fairly self-explanatory. Do not forget to familiarize yourself with the labeling controls, in particular the left and right orientation for parasagittal images.

Care of the baby during scanning
Risks

Sick premature neonates can be very unstable, and so accommodation of certain factors must be considered when proposing cranial ultrasound. The greatest risk during scanning a premature baby is that of the procedure, which increases handling the baby, causing discomfort and stress. The effects range from a brief period of crying and distress, to an accidental extubation of intubated ventilated infants. It is easy to underestimate the harm that can be done by inappropriate scanning!

Time

Try to take as little time as possible in order to keep the baby stable, especially if they are in an incubator. Make an effort to minimize environmental disturbances, such as ambient heat, humidity, noise and even ambient oxygen level changes. Most scans should be limited to a maximum of 10 min, frequently requiring much less time than this.

Sedation

Sedation is rarely required. Good restraint can be obtained (if necessary) from nursing support, wrapping the baby in a blanket, just after a good feed, or a combination of these. A sleeping baby is the ideal subject, although it is not necessary for the baby to be stationary, or for the head to be in the midline, as the transducer probe can be moved easily with the baby – do not try to resist movement! Ideally, the probe should not move from the anterior fontanelle (the maximal acoustic window) during scanning, else signal dropout becomes obvious – it may be necessary to reposition the probe repeatedly, or rest a finger on the baby's head to keep the probe in position. Oxygen saturations and heart rate should be monitored throughout. This makes ultrasound particularly suitable for this cohort of patients who may not be stable enough to be transported to a CT or MRI scanner.

Consent

Departments will have their own policy regarding informed consent. Currently it is thought that parental consent is no longer considered as implied, and therefore verbal, if not written, consent *should* be sought before undertaking each procedure. It is generally considered *not* appropriate to have parents present at scanning, in case of misinterpretation of pathology, or the sudden appearance of obvious pathology with a very poor prognosis. All scans need to be reviewed by the team, so it is essential to keep a recording. It is unwise to give parents an instant diagnosis at the time of scan, in lieu of reviewing the recording with a more experienced operator.

Infection

There are nosocomial infection control implications in scanning multiple babies with the same probe, or even with the same gel tube. Cleaning the probe using alcohol between scans and rigorous hand washing between patients will reduce infection risks, as will the use of sterile gel from individual sachets. The probe may be covered with a layer of sterile dressing such as Tegaderm, provided that

air bubbles are excluded. It is good practice to use individual packets of gel.

Heat production

There is the theoretical risk of local heat production during ultrasound scanning, although there is currently no evidence of any harm to patients. Conventional 2D scanning produces very small changes in thermal heat with minimal risk, but using Doppler imaging increases the output and concentrates the beam on a much smaller area, and so its use should be kept to a minimum and only when clinically necessary.

When to scan

The best time to scan a well neonate remains controversial, and may depend on pragmatic and practical factors rather than clinical ones. The minimum should be at least one scan during the first week of life, to detect early pathology; one during the second week of life to look for progression; and one "late" scan at 4–6 weeks of age, to check for sequelae and missed pathology. Most units would advocate a comprehensive scan during the first 24–48 h, and if there are any abnormalities, alternate days for the first 7 days, and fortnightly thereafter until discharge. More frequent scanning may be dictated by clinical condition. Routine cranial ultrasound is currently recommended for all babies born before 32 weeks, due to the increased susceptibility to the pathologies described here.

Standard scanning planes

Scanning is conventionally done through the anterior fontanelle, although the posterior fontanelle and any widely separated skull sutures will allow similar access. By placing the probe at the anterior fontanelle, two distinct planes are readily accessible: coronal and sagittal planes (Figures 10.1 and 10.2). Axial planes are not routinely used in neonatal scanning. Holding the probe with the operator's

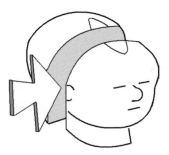

Figure 10.1 Direction of coronal view.

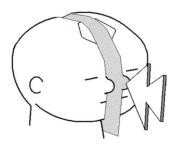

Figure 10.2 Direction of sagittal view.

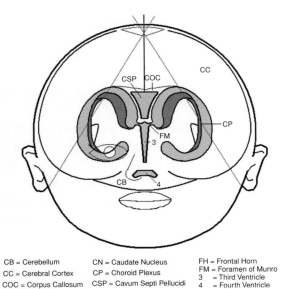

CB = Cerebellum	CN = Caudate Nucleus	FH = Frontal Horn
CC = Cerebral Cortex	CP = Choroid Plexus	FM = Foramen of Munro
COC = Corpus Callosum	CSP = Cavum Septi Pellucidi	3 = Third Ventricle
		4 = Fourth Ventricle

Figure 10.3 Diagrammatic representation of standard coronal view.

dominant hand allows the cord to be supported over the shoulders, to take the weight from the back of the probe. Remember that it is easier to break the cable than the probe, at a significant cost.

The convention is to determine the coronal midline image (frontal view; Figure 10.3), sweeping as far anteriorly and then posteriorly as possible, then rotating the probe to identify the midline sagittal image (anterior–posterior view; Figure 10.8), and sweeping as far laterally (left and right view) as possible. The scan operator then goes back to record the scan, if they have not already done so, and to print freeze-frame images. There are six standard images that are the "minimum required" to constitute a successful scan: coronal midline, anterior oblique coronal, posterior oblique coronal, midline sagittal, left and right parasagittal.

Coronal plane

Start by identifying the midline coronal view (Figure 10.3). Most probes will have a notch or marker on one side, which should be directed to the patient's left side, to help identify the patient's left on the scan. The midline view cuts through both ventricles, corpus callosum and basal ganglia (Figure 10.5, on DVD). Use the symmetry of the Sylvian fissures to assess the probe's symmetry, and scan quickly to one side to confirm that your designation of left and right is in fact correct.

Sweep anteriorly to examine the anterior brain parenchyma, anterior to the frontal horns of the lateral ventricles (Figure 10.4, on DVD). Sweep posteriorly to the back of the ventricles, going through the level of the third ventricle, thalami and choroid plexi (Figure 10.6, on DVD). Finally, check the posterior brain parenchyma, posterior to the posterior horns of the lateral ventricles (Figure 10.7, on DVD), and finally the cerebellar region. Remember that these are not true coronal scans, but are oblique coronal views through the anterior fontanelle.

Sagittal plane

By rotating the probe through 90°, the midline sagittal view can be delineated (Figure 10.8). Neither lateral ventricle should be seen in the midline,

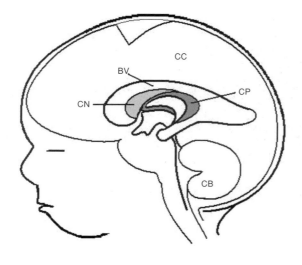

BV = Body of ventricle
CB = Cerebellum
CC = Cerebral cortex
CN = Caudate nucleus
CP = Choroid plexus

Figure 10.8 Diagrammatic representation of standard sagittal view.

but the cavum septum pellucidum, cerebellar region and occasionally the third ventricle can be seen (Figure 10.9, on DVD). The corpus callosum should be seen in the midline. Sweep one side through the ventricles to look for abnormal size and content, particularly in the occipital horns of the lateral ventricles (parasagittal view; Figure 10.10, on DVD), and check for extension into the cortex beyond the ventricular system. The germinal matrix is of particular importance in the neonate. The choroid plexus appears bright at the posterior aspect and can resemble hemorrhage to the inexperienced user. Always sweep lateral to the lateral ventricles to identify the lateral brain parenchyma (Figure 10.11, on DVD), including the sulcal and gyral pattern, and then return to the midline in order to repeat this process for the opposite side. Remember to mark the left and right sagittal views on the screen for recording, otherwise it is impossible to tell which side is which. Remember that the lateral ventricles do not run exactly anterior–

posterior: instead, they tend to run antero-lateral to postero-medial.

Work through the layers of tissue to identify the presence of pathology or absence of structures, using this guide as a checklist. Always remember that changes need to be seen in both coronal and sagittal planes.

(1) Identify the presence, symmetry and overall size of lateral ventricles, as well as the third and fourth ventricles.
(2) Check the germinal matrix, and choroid plexuses, and try to identify if there is any extra tissue in the ventricular system which could be hemorrhage.
(3) Identify the presence of the corpus callosum (along the entire midline sagittal view). If the corpus callosum is aplastic or absent, the lateral ventricles will be pulled into the midline.
(4) Check the entire cortex for normal parenchymal appearances.
(5) Check the cerebellar parenchyma for gross abnormalities.
(6) If pathology is present, is it unilateral or bilateral?
(7) Is there one lesion or more than one, and are they related?
(8) Check whether the gyral and sulcal pattern is abnormal or gestation-appropriate?
(9) If the ventricles appear dilated, they can be measured and referred to normal values.

Practical limitations to scanning include the width of the probe in comparison to the size of the fontanelle, although a standard size should do.

Frequently encountered errors

There are a number of errors which occur in scans performed by inexperienced operators, and these can be mostly avoided by following some key principles

(1) It is better to have a generous amount rather than insufficient gel for image quality, although beware the probe may slip off with excess gel!

(2) Scanning may be limited by the size of the fontanelle, but gentle pressure applied to the probe on the fontanelle should increase the scanning window to allow adequate assessment.

(3) Remember to scan to the proximities in every plane, in order not to miss superficial lesions.

(4) There is frequently signal drop-out at the extremities of the scanning plane, particularly very anteriorly and very posteriorly; in order not to miss superficial lesions, the probe may need to be re-positioned slightly to visualize all areas and structures.

(5) If the image is too dark (incorrect contrast set/receiver gain), then parenchymal lesions may be missed due to insufficient differentiation.

(6) If the image is too bright (incorrect contrast set/receiver gain), parenchymal echodensities may be overdiagnosed.

These points emphasize the need for a senior member of the team to review the scan prior to a report being given.

Indications for use

Premature babies are the commonest subjects requiring cranial ultrasound scans, as they have particularly good fontanelle access, and are particularly at risk of severe hemorrhage. Scans can be performed up to 6–9 months of age, or until the fontanelle closes.

Ultrasound is used to diagnose intraventricular hemorrhage, but is less good at identifying extradural and subdural hemorrhages, which are too close to the surface. Pathology that can be identified can be broadly classified into the following.

(1) Intraventricular and periventricular hemorrhage.

(2) Hydrocephalus and ventricular dilatation, with or without hemorrhage. Serial scans assist in making ventricular measurements (see cases below) and planning surgery.

(3) White matter injury, typically periventricular leucomalacia (PVL).

(4) Developmental abnormalities, which may be:
   (a) cerebellar, such as Dandy Walker malformations,
   (b) cortical, such as pachygyri and lissencephaly, or
   (c) midline structures, such as agenesis of the corpus callosum.

(5) Intracranial calcification – particularly with congenital infection, such as toxoplasmosis or cytomegalovirus (CMV).

(6) Other rarer pathologies, such as neonatal tumors and cerebral ischemia.

Doppler ultrasound

Doppler ultrasound measures blood flow velocity, although there are few clinical situations when it is specifically needed. The velocity of cerebral blood flow in neonates, in the main intracerebral vessels, increases both with gestational age and post-natal age, such that the lower resistance at lower gestational ages may explain the greater susceptibility to intracerebral hemorrhages of the immature infant. There are a large number of variables that can affect blood flow velocity, including: posture, sleep, medication, arterial carbon dioxide and oxygen levels, and the presence of cardiac lesions (such as a patent ductus arteriosus), such that it is not a reliable measure. It can be used to demonstrate turbulent flow in a vein of Galen aneurysm, and has been used to assess outcome in neonates with hypoxic ischemic encephalopathy. Given the safety issues mentioned, the consensus is that most clinical questions can be answered without the use of Doppler scanning, and thus its use should be minimal and caution used in its interpretation, except in infants with hypoxic ischemic encephalopathy.

Illustrative case histories with example scans

Case 1

A premature baby is born in good condition at 29 weeks gestation to a Caucasian mother aged 18 years. The baby is well, ventilated for a short time only, and receives routine neonatal care, remaining clinically well for the first week of life. A routine cranial ultrasound was performed.

The ultrasound scan shows a small echodense lesion on top of the choroid plexus, characteristically at the caudo-thalamic groove (Figures 10.12 and 10.13, both on DVD). This is a germinal matrix hemorrhage (GMH), the simplest type of intraventricular hemorrhage seen, also known as Grade I (Table 10.1). It may be difficult to differentiate from so-called "bulky" choroids (of no prognostic significance), and serial scans may be required to determine the nature of this lesion.

The germinal matrix is a site of neuronal proliferation as neuroblasts divide and migrate into the cerebral parenchyma, with neuronal proliferation complete by 20 weeks gestation, and glial cell proliferation complete around 32 weeks gestation. The germinal matrix involutes thereafter, and is usually not identifiable after 36 weeks gestation. Cells of the germinal matrix are rich in mitochondria and therefore quite sensitive to ischemia. Most intraventricular hemorrhages of this type occur because of hypoxia–ischemia reperfusion injury to the very fragile vascular bed at this particular area. For these reasons, intraventricular hemorrhages (IVHs) are common in preterm infants, but unusual beyond 32–33 weeks gestational age.

GMHs occur at the caudo-thalamic groove; they may be entirely asymptomatic, and may have no prognostic significance. They may extend to form intraventricular hemorrhages, may resolve and disappear completely, or may develop an echolucent cystic center which degenerates into a subependymal pseudocyst (SEPC). These may also be seen during the first few days of life, indicating an antenatal event giving rise to a GMH, such as intrauterine infection or maternal drug abuse.

Case 2

A premature baby is born in good condition at 25 weeks gestation to a young mother. His APGAR score at birth is 3 at 1 min and 7 at 5 min of age. He is intubated and given a dose of surfactant and is transferred to a neonatal intensive care unit. The baby requires intermittent positive pressure ventilation, but becomes stable on the ventilator. At 6 h of age, there is a sudden deterioration in the baby's respiratory condition, with profound acidosis and hypoxia that appears unrelated to ventilator settings. A cranial ultrasound is requested.

Figures 10.14 and 10.15 (both on DVD) show an echodense blood clot in both lateral ventricles on coronal view. These represent bilateral IVHs (Grade II). Intraventricular hemorrhages are the commonest lesion detected by cranial ultrasound, and the commonest important cause of long-term neurodisability (Table 10.1). The risk of any type of IVH decreases significantly with increasing gestational age. Fifty per cent of GMH/IVHs will occur in the first 6–8 h of life, and the vast majority (over 90%) occur within 3 days. IVHs may also resolve completely, may give mild persistent ventricular dilatation of limited significance, or the blood may obstruct CSF flow, and thus eventually hydrocephalus with gross ventricular dilatation (Grade III; Figure 10.16, on DVD).

A GMH or IVH may obstruct the draining veins in the region of the germinal matrix, which may cause a venous infarct. This is called a hemorrhagic parenchymal infarct (HPI, or Grade IV IVH; Figure 10.17, on DVD) to differentiate from periventricular ischemia, which is arterial in origin. HPI gives rise to wedge-shaped echodense lesions extending from the lateral border of the lateral ventricle into the parenchyma. These lesions were previously thought to be actual hemorrhage "extending" into the parenchyma from the ventricle, but are now

Table 10.1 Traditional categorization of periventricular hemorrhages (after Papile *et al.*, 1978).

Grade	Also called	Highest estimated mortality	Prognosis	Risk of subsequent disability*	What happens if lesion progresses
I	Isolated Germinal matrix haemorrhage (GMH)	<10%	Excellent "low risk"	10–30%	May give rise to HPI May extend into IVH May regress into SEPC
II	Isolated Intraventricular hemorrhage (IVH)	30%	Usually good "moderate risk"	10–50%	May develop PHHC May give rise to HPI
III	Intraventricular hemorrhage with ventricular dilatation	60%	Usually poor "high risk"	25–60%	May develop PHHC May give rise to HPI
IV	IVH with HPI – Hemorrhagic parenchymal infarct	90%	Usually poor "high risk"	60–80%	May regress into PEC

This classification suggests progression from Grades I to IV, which is now recognized not to occur in all cases. Whilst a GMH may progress to an IVH and then cause ventricular expansion, Grade II can exist without Grade I, and it is clear that hemorrhagic parenchymal infarcts (HPIs) can occur without intraventricular hemorrhage. Grades I and II account for around 75% of all IVHs
*Note: risk of disability of all preterm infants with no GMH/IVH is around 10%.
Abbreviations used: GMH: germinal matrix hemorrhage; IVH: intraventricular hemorrhage; HPI: hemorrhagic parenchymal infarct; SEPC: subependymal pseudocyst; PEC: porencephalic cyst.

known to occur with minimal hemorrhage, due to venous obstruction. HPIs are usually unilateral, and appear within the first few days of life. They may resolve to leave a single cystic lesion in continuity with the lateral ventricle, known as a porencephalic cyst (PeC). HPIs are nearly always associated with a contralateral hemiplegia, although overall intellectual development may be preserved in unilateral insults, sometimes even despite large loss of brain tissue.

Case 3

A baby is born at 29 weeks gestation by emergency cesarean section to a 30-year-old mother. There was antenatal intrauterine growth restriction and fetal distress for an hour prior to delivery. The baby requires resuscitation at birth and has poor blood gas readings initially, although these improve. An initial ultrasound shows bilateral intraventricular hemorrhages. The baby is scanned serially over the first few days of life, and an increasing head circumference is noted. A repeat cranial ultrasound on day 7 is requested. In this case, hemorrhage in the ventricles has impeded the normal absorption of CSF through the arachnoid villi, leading to CSF accumulation (Figures 10.18 and 10.19, both on DVD).

Ventricular width (previously called ventricular index, or VI, in millimeters) may be measured as the horizontal distance across the widest point of the lateral ventricles, on a coronal image on which both foramina of Munro and the third ventricle are visible. There are gestation-dependent standards (approximately 9 mm at 28 weeks, to 12 mm at 40 weeks). Another commonly used method for grading hydrocephalus is the ventricular/hemispheric (V/H) ratio. It is ideally taken at the level of foramen of Monro/third ventricle in coronal section. The distance of the lateral wall of the lateral ventricle from midline to the hemispheric width, if more than 0.35, is suggestive of ventricular enlargement.

When considering ventricular dilatation, it is important to consider different pathological causes, particularly progressive dilatation secondary to increased intraventricular fluid or obstruction (increased intraventricular pressure), versus ventricular dilatation due to surrounding cerebral atrophy (normal intraventricular pressure). In the former, the ventricular walls are smooth and the enlargement is typically rapid, associated with increasing head circumference; whereas in the latter, the ventricular walls are typically irregular with no enlargement of head circumference, and slow enlargement of the ventricles. Serial ultrasound scans are particularly useful in following the progression of these lesions.

There are numerous other causes of ventricular enlargement in the perinatal period, with congenital abnormalities, such as aqueductal stenosis, and congenital infection causing ventriculitis, being common. Often hydrocephalus can be diagnosed antenatally, in which cases associated CNS/extracranial anomalies should be looked for, particularly meningomyeloceles and other neural tube defects.

Although 50% of neonatal hydrocephalus may resolve spontaneously, definitive management of ventricular enlargement under pressure is that of a surgical ventricular reservoir or ventriculo-peritoneal shunt. Lytic agents such as streptokinase have also been used to breakdown clots causing hydrocephalus, but within minimal benefit. Children with hydrocephalus may suffer no adverse neurodevelopmental consequences; those who develop post-hemorrhagic hydrocephalus are typically associated with an poorer outcome.

Case 4

A baby is born at 28 weeks gestation with severe intrauterine growth restriction, and required resuscitation following delivery. He was ventilated for 72 h but made good progress and was spontaneously ventilating in air by 5 days of age. Initial routine cranial ultrasounds scans are reported as normal, but it is noted that the baby has reduced power and increased tone in its left arm and leg. As the hemiplegia does not recover, a repeat cranial ultrasound is performed at 8 weeks of age, showing periventricular leucomalacia (PVL; Figures 10.20 and 10.21, both on DVD).

Ultrasound is much less sensitive at detecting ischemic lesions as compared to hemorrhagic lesions, particularly in the early stages. Early changes of ischemia are seen as slight echodensity, or "flare", within the periventricular white matter. The main concern with these lesions is that, with time, if they do not resolve completely, they may progress to leave multiple, frequently large cystic (echolucent) lesions, termed periventricular leucomalacia (PVL). These cysts are *not* in communication with the ventricles, unlike the porencephalic cysts which follow resolving HPIs. PVL seen in the first few days of life therefore indicates antenatal ischemia, commonly due to ante-partum hemorrhage, maternal trauma, or infection.

To distinguish ischemic white matter from normal parenchymal tissue is not easy using ultrasound techniques, although some diagnostic criteria have been suggested. Ischemia should have the following typical characteristics.

(a) Involving white matter adjacent to the ventricles.
(b) Being at least as bright as the choroids plexuses (in case of poor gain settings).
(c) Not being associated with intraventricular hemorrhage (although they may co-exist).
(d) Not being well-defined (in contrast to wedge-shaped venous infarcts/HPI).

These changes are subtle and serial scans are required to track the progression of the lesion to confirm a doubtful diagnosis. There is frequently a delay between a neurological insult and the appearance of lesions, as normal appearances may be seen up to 6–8 weeks post-delivery, but subsequently show significant white matter lesions. This suggests exercising caution when reassuring parents regarding normal early scans, which may subsequently reveal gross lesions with significant morbidity.

PVL subsequently degenerates into multiple small and discrete cysts, being distinct rather than coalescing with the ventricles (cf. porencephalic cysts). Both hemorrhagic and ischemic lesions may occur simultaneously, although the pathophysiology is different. The pathophysiology of PVL is likely to be multifactorial, involving both so-called watershed injury (the border zones of deep penetrating arteries of the middle cerebral artery) to the periventricular area due to a vascular insult, and/or maternal chorioamnionitis or vasculitis, leading to inflammatory cytokine-mediated damage.

Decreased blood flow affects the white matter at the supero-lateral borders of the lateral ventricles. The site of injury affects the descending corticospinal tracts, visual radiations, and acoustic radiations. Premature infants on mechanical ventilation may develop hypocarbia, which has been linked with the development of PVL. In addition to possible ischemic injury, PVL may be the result of edema fluid and hemorrhage causing compression of arterioles in the white matter. Premature infants have impaired cerebrovascular autoregulation and are susceptible to intracranial hemorrhage (ICH) as well as PVL. Many premature infants have both PVL and ICH detected on ultrasonography.

The presence of PVL is usually associated with clinical morbidity, and is predominantly associated with very low birth weight infants (<1500 g). Around 60–80% of infants with PVL later develop signs of cerebral palsy, and some will develop varying degrees of intellectual impairment, developmental impairment, and visual dysfunction. Small lesions may resolve to leave non-detectable pathology or morbidity, whereas extensive lesions may coalesce and cause more global neurodevelopmental insult. The specific location of periventricular cystic damage may have some prognostic significance: descending tracts from motor cortex (particularly lower limbs) are generally located superior and lateral to the LVs, and so PVL in these areas is typically linked to development of spastic diplegia. Severe PVL is frequently associated with quadriplegia. The prognosis is frequently proportional to the extent and severity of PVL, with the "worst" scan being the "most" prognostic, but not always.

Case 5

A baby is born at term but has a cleft palate, and hypoplasia of its mid-facial features. A cranial ultrasound is requested in case of further intracranial midline abnormalities. An echolucent area is seen on coronal scanning at the base of the brain within the posterior fossa. The Dandy Walker complex (Figures 10.22 and 10.23, both on DVD) is a cystic abnormality consisting of an enlarged posterior fossa, complete or partial agenesis of the cerebellar vermis, massive dilatation of the fourth ventricle filling the posterior fossa, and hydrocephalus (which may not occur until later). This complex may present later with increasing head circumference, or developmental delay. Neurodevelopmental outcomes are extremely variable. It accounts for around 10% of cases of congenital hydrocephalus. Other, more common causes of hydrocephalus include aqueductal stenosis and Arnold Chiari malformations (inferior displacement of cerebellar tonsils).

Case 6

A 3-month-old boy was brought in from home by ambulance to the emergency department. The baby had been found blue and lifeless on the floor that morning, after the father had fallen asleep on the sofa with the baby in his arms. There was no past medical history of note, and the baby had been well the previous night. The baby had been successfully resuscitated by the paramedics, and on arrival was breathing spontaneously but with a depressed conscious level. Unfortunately, there were no CT scanning facilities at the admitting hospital, but a rapid cranial ultrasound by the pediatric registrar in the emergency department showed large bilateral intraventricular hemorrhages, similar to those of Figure 10.14, on DVD. There was also the suggestion of a subdural bleed. The baby was ventilated for transfer to a hospital with suitable intensive care and neurosurgical facilities. Subsequent X-rays of the long bones showed an old spiral fracture of the femur and multiple posterior rib fractures. These injuries are characteristic of non-accidental injury, particularly with multiple injuries of different ages at different sites.

Other pathology

Ultrasound can also frequently demonstrate other pathology. The operator should ensure that the corpus callosum is identified throughout its entire length, as there are many conditions associated with defects in, or total agenesis of, the corpus callosum. The incidental finding of intracranial calcification (calcium appears bright white, similar to bone, on an ultrasound scan) is unusual, but is most commonly associated with the transplacental passage of viral infections during pregnancy, which may have been asymptomatic. Scattered and subependymal intracranial calcification is typically seen following intrauterine toxoplasmosis infection, whereas periventricular intracranial calcification is typically seen following intrauterine cytomegalovirus infection. Intrauterine HIV can also cause intracranial calcification, particularly in the basal ganglia. However, these diseases should not be differentiated by the pattern of intracranial infection alone, and sonographic findings must always be taken in the context of the neonatal clinical presentation.

Limitations

Whilst cranial ultrasound is strong in certain areas, other areas are notably weaker. These include anatomical constraints, such as when the anterior fontanelles close (between 9 and 18 months; the posterior fontanelle closes around 3 months), and

problems of penetration, such that the posterior fossa is relatively inaccessible with high-frequency scanning.

Many structural lesions will be clearly visualized by real-time ultrasound, though these are likely to be confirmed by further neuroimaging (CT or MRI) later. Some areas of the brain are less accessible to ultrasound, including the posterior fossa and brainstem, although the range of pathologies that can be identified early on include Dandy Walker malformations, Arnold Chiari, cerebellar hypoplasia, and agenesis of the corpus callosum.

Ultrasound has a limited role in birth asphyxia, now correctly called "hypoxic ischemic encephalopathy" (HIE), and other forms of neonatal encephalopathy. The brain may appear brighter than normal within the first week, often with sparing of the thalamus and cerebellum, and subsequently the ventricles become "slit-like" structures. Later scans may show evidence of cerebral atrophy and enlarged ventricles. However, as none of these features are pathognomonic, MRI is now the dominant imaging modality of choice in these types of diffuse white matter pathology.

By categorizing lesions seen on ultrasound, useful information can be obtained about the likelihood of long-term neurodevelopmental impairment. However, diagnostic scan results should be interpreted with caution and in the light of the clinical picture. A normal or low-risk scan, while reassuring, is not always associated with a normal neurodevelopmental outcome; conversely, a small proportion of infants with high-risk scans will have little or no associated neurodisability. However, infants at significant risk of disability can be identified early and can be referred early for detailed surveillance, targeted therapy and educational help.

Conclusions

Neonatal cranial ultrasound scanning is a valuable tool in the management of the preterm infant.

It can be seen as a screening tool for the vast majority of preterm babies, and for identifying major abnormalities in term babies. There are diagnostic difficulties, both machine-dependent, and operator-dependent. In the majority of cases where significant abnormalities are seen, particularly with regard to the posterior fossa and parenchymal abnormalities, serial scanning and sometimes more definitive imaging will be required. This does not limit ultrasound's usefulness; rather, it creates a domain for rapid, safe, non-invasive, repeatable imaging in the critically sick neonate, which may be inaccessible by other means.

Acknowledgments

With thanks to Dr. Wilf Kelsall, Neonatal Intensive Care Unit, Cambridge, for helpful advice on the preparation of this manuscript. The author is also grateful to Tony Bailey for the line illustrations.

FURTHER READING

Rennie JM. *Neonatal Cerebral Ultrasound*. Cambridge, Cambridge University Press 1997.

Govaert G, de Vries LS. *An Atlas of Neonatal Brain Sonography*. Cambridge, Cambridge University Press 1997.

Rennie JM. *Roberton's Textbook of Neonatology*, 4th edn. New York, Churchill Livingstone, 2005.

American Institute of Ultrasound Medicine. *Guidelines for the Performance of the Pediatric Neurosonology Ultrasound Examination*. Rockville: American Institute of Ultrasound Medicine, 1991.

Papile LA, Burnstein J, Burnstein R, Koffler H. Incidence and evolution of subependymal and intraventricular hemorrhage: a study of infants with birth weights less than 1,500 gm. *Journal of Pediatrics* 1978;92:529–34.

Chapter **11**

The use of ultrasound in acute gynecology and pregnancy assessment

WILLIAM TAYLOR

Introduction

In 1958 a landmark case established ultrasound as an important medical tool. This was the use by Ian Donald of ultrasound to diagnose an easily removable ovarian cyst, which had previously been thought to be an inoperable stomach tumor.

Ultrasound is now established as an essential diagnostic tool in obstetrics and gynecology. Ultrasound examination complements clinical history taking and examination, but does not replace it.

The majority of imaging in gynecology and early pregnancy is transvaginal by virtue of the greatly improved image quality it provides. The sonographer should be sensitive to the layout of the scanning room and the patient not positioned facing the door unless it is screened. All staff should be chaperoned when performing intimate examinations on patients. Transvaginal scanning is best achieved using a couch specifically designed for the purpose with the patient's legs supported in a low modified lithotomy position (Figures 11.1 and 11.2, both on DVD). If a conventional examination couch is used, a pillow is placed under the patient's buttocks and the legs supported at the end of an examination couch (Figure 11.3, on DVD). The patient's bladder is emptied prior to the examination, but some operators prefer to have a small fluid residue in the bladder to provide an anatomical reference point. The

operator wears gloves and should enquire about latex allergy prior to sheathing the ultrasound probe (Figure 11.4, on DVD). The probe is introduced in the same manner as a vaginal speculum. The vaginal probe and orientation of scanning is less related to anatomical planes since the axis of the uterus seldom lies completely in the midline and the ovaries may be extremely mobile. Most women have an anteverted uterus and the cervix will consequently be directed posteriorly in the vagina. This should be the starting position for the probe. Once the uterus is identified, the probe is either rotated slightly or moved to one side or the other to orientate with the long axis of the uterus and then lifted up or down to include the uterine fundus in the image. Distortion of the image is normal on transvaginal scanning and produces a banana-shaped uterus even when clinical examination shows it is clearly straight (Figure 11.5, on DVD). This distortion is due to the small transducer surface on a vaginal probe and the curvature of the array. The ultrasound beam arises as a fan from the transducer surface, and the image structures so generated appear to wrap around the transducer on the screen (Figure 11.6, on DVD).

There must be room to maneuver the probe handle down into the couch to complete the field of view. This is particularly important when trying

Ultrasound in Anesthetic Practice, ed. Graham Arthurs and Barry Nicholls. Published by Cambridge University Press.
© Cambridge University Press 2009.

158

to locate the ovaries. To identify the ovaries, commence at the uterine fundus, move laterally to one or other cornu and the adnexa commences at this point. A lateral sweep should then identify the ovary since it is held from this area by a suspensory ligament. If unsuccessful, then the next region to search is posterior to the uterus as at times the ovaries fall into the Pouch of Douglas. Occasionally, if the woman has had previous surgery, adhesions may pull an ovary up from the pelvis. Bowel gas may obscure the view even with transvaginal scanning; hence locating normal ovaries is not always a certainty (Figure 11.7, on DVD).

Transabdominal scanning requires a full bladder. This is to facilitate imaging since the fluid-filled bladder transmits sound directly down to the uterus and also for anatomical reference. Shadowing from bowel gas is more problematic and asking the women to roll over to one or other side may move bowel and improve imaging. This maneuver is also useful later in pregnancy when the fetus may obscure imaging of a posterior placenta. Alternatively, rotation of the fetus may improve viewing of the face or heart. In late pregnancy a full bladder is largely irrelevant for fetal imaging, unless used as a reference point for a low placental edge. Transabdominal transducers typically have a marker on the probe casing for orientation (Figure 11.8, on DVD). There are two possible layouts for equipment when scanning abdominally. Conventionally, the operator faces the patient and the screen, with the latter facing away from the patient. Alternatively, the ultrasound machine may be placed at the woman's feet and both patient and operator face in the same direction towards the screen. It depends on preference and the purpose of the examination.

Ultrasound in obstetrics with acute gynecology
Non-obstetric complications of pregnancy
Much of acute gynecological practice includes the complications of pregnancy. A pregnancy test prior to ultrasound examination is essential. Ultrasound is a useful tool in the assessment of abdominal or pelvic pain.

Threatened miscarriage and early pregnancy
The modern over-the-counter pregnancy test is both sensitive and specific. Biochemical diagnosis is possible at the time of the missed period or within days of it occurring and before anything is visible on ultrasound scanning. At 5 weeks with optimal transvaginal scanning, a 10 mm gestation sac may be visible, but it may give no more information. A fetal pole may appear at 6 weeks, and a heart beat at 7 weeks (Figures 11.9a, 11.9b); thereafter, the fetus becomes recognizable as such. The yolk sac may be visible before the fetus, and may be the marker of an ongoing pregnancy prior to the later appearance of

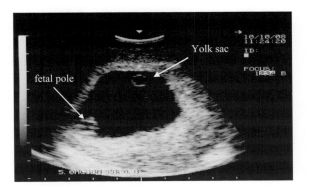

Figure 11.9a Seven-week gestation.

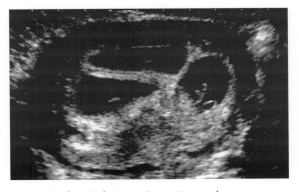

Figure 11.9b Triplet gestation at 7+ weeks.

the fetal heart. Transvaginal scanning (TVS) is the standard approach prior to 10 weeks amenorrhea as transabdominal scanning, even with a full bladder, may not give adequate definition, particularly with a high body mass index (BMI). After 10 weeks an adequate image is obtained by transabdominal scanning with a full bladder to be able to identify fetal parts (Figure 11.10, on DVD).

Scanning women with threatened miscarriage is principally concerned with establishing fetal viability.

Case history of bleeding in early pregnancy

A 28-year-old lady presented at 14 weeks amenorrhea with painful vaginal bleeding. The uterine fundus was just palpable by abdominal examination and a fetal heartbeat was audible with sonicaid. The ultrasound findings were of a twin pregnancy and bleeding was due to the demise of one fetus (Figure 11.11, on DVD). It was a dichorionic diamniotic twin pregnancy (non-identical with separate sacs) and the smaller twin on the left seen in longitudinal section is dead. Measurement gave crown–rump length (CRL) 46.4 mm (11 weeks 3 days), whereas the viable twin seen only in transverse section had a bi-parietal diameter (BPD) of 25.9 mm (14 weeks 1 day).

Many more pregnancies commence as twin than complete as such. The UK rate is currently 1 in 80 deliveries. The incidence has been rising in recent years due to assisted conception (IVF).

Early diagnosis of twins, where both are viable, is important for planning antenatal care and chorionicity (configuration of membranes) is related to subsequent morbidity. The lambda sign, "Y", shows the presence of placental tissue between gestation sacs (Figure 11.12, on DVD). This is diagnostic of a dichorionic, diamniotic twin gestation – two sacs each with its own separate chorion and amnion, whereas its absence (Figure 11.13, on DVD) suggests a single chorion.

Ectopic pregnancy

Early intra-uterine pregnancy failure is seldom life-threatening, but ectopic pregnancy is important. The classical clinical picture of an ectopic gestation is 7 weeks amenorrhea with pelvic pain and vaginal bleeding. Sometimes there is syncope and shoulder tip pain. The dilemma with early biochemical confirmation of pregnancy and vague clinical symptoms is that ultrasound signs may initially be absent or subtle. Initially there may be a slight thickening of the endometrium, or a rim of fluid around the uterus or Pouch of Douglas. A pseudo sac within the endometrium may mislead the operator. The margins of the sac, however, are indistinct and represent an endometrial reaction, which never develops further. Later the free fluid will be apparent, and there is development of a cystic mass in one of the adnexae. Very occasionally a gestation sac is visible outside of the uterus. Any one of these signs in the context of clinical suspicion, with a positive pregnancy test and with no visible sign of a gestation with the uterus, raises the possibility of a diagnosis of ectopic pregnancy.

Case history of ectopic gestation

This case presented with persistent abdominal pain at 7 weeks amenorrhea, minimal bleeding and a positive pregnancy test (Figure 11.14, on DVD). On transvaginal scanning, the uterus is empty with a defined midline echo. There is substantial free fluid in the Pouch of Douglas to the right and also anteriorly between the uterus and the bladder. In the context of the history, this is almost certainly blood. The partially filled bladder is just visible top left. The gestation sac became visible only on turning the probe laterally to visualize the adnexa, and is seen not in the salpinx but is sited in the left cornu, and could have been missed from the initial image (Figure 11.15, on DVD). Further movement of the probe laterally isolates the image of the gestation. Note the salpinx itself is not visualized and is not seen unless defined by fluid either distending it or surrounding it (Figure 11.16, on DVD).

Case history of mild ovarian hyperstimulation

Fertility treatment is commonplace in gynecological practice and occasionally ovarian hyperstimulation may present with abdominal pain accompanied by vomiting.

A lady of 34 years underwent her first stimulated ovarian cycle and conceived successfully. There was some abdominal pain in the first few weeks of pregnancy, which flared up as an acute abdomen with right iliac fossa pain at 12 weeks gestation. There was no vaginal bleeding. There was no pyrexia or cardiovascular shock. Hematological and biochemical tests were normal. Ultrasound examination confirmed a viable 12 week gestation fetus and free fluid in the pelvis. A follow up scan 5 days after presentation, when transabdominal scanning was more comfortable, showed an enlarged right ovary with residual follicles (Figure 11.17, on DVD). The symptoms settled with conservative treatment.

Pathology co-existing with pregnancy

Apart from the functional corpus luteum, ovarian cysts may predate pregnancy and, being fluid-filled, may enlarge progressively with hormone stimulation. Blood vessels may be disrupted by capsular growth producing hemorrhage within the cyst (Figure 11.18, on DVD). Hemorrhage is seen as a semi-solid mass within the cyst, which may produce particulate matter, and in the acute phase. Transducer pressure may aggravate the pain. Free fluid in the peritoneum is unlikely. The image illustrates a pre-existing cyst where pregnancy occurred prior to the intended treatment. Hospital admission was required and ultrasound scanning demonstrated cyst enlargement (117×83 mm). The area of hemorrhage within the cyst had a cross-sectional area of 59×38 mm. The acute abdomen, which resulted, required laparotomy, but the pregnancy remained viable.

Gynecology
Pelvic inflammatory disease

Salpingitis presenting for the first time may be seen as an adnexal mass (pyosalpinx) with a small amount of free fluid around the adnexa or uterus. The normal Fallopian tube is not visible on ultrasound scanning, and appears only when the presence of fluid either within it or around it enhances its appearance. Pelvic inflammatory disease (PID), which becomes a more chronic condition, shows fewer ultrasound signs. Often tissues are sensitive and the ultrasound probe can trigger localized pain, and fibrosed tissue shows less or no movement with respiration or bodily movement.

Endometriosis

This occasionally presents as acute pelvic pain. The classical signs of match-head sized inflammatory deposits of endometriosis are beyond the resolution of ultrasound imaging, but the ovaries may exhibit collections of hemorrhage within the stroma – typically endometriomas. The utero-sacral ligaments may show thickening and the uterine myometrium can show deposits similar to the ovaries, particularly in parous women. These tissues may show restricted movement and tenderness on transvaginal scanning.

Ultrasound in normal obstetrics
THE DATING SCAN

In antenatal care, often the first point of contact with the hospital is the dating scan appointment. It is crucial to the screening process to accurately date the pregnancy. Modern over-the-counter pregnancy kits are so sensitive (positive at 25–30 IU hcg) that the biochemical diagnosis of pregnancy is made before anything is visible by ultrasound. For early ultrasound imaging of pregnancy before 10 weeks, transvaginal scanning (TVS) is the norm.

The first opportunity to visualize an intra-uterine gestation sac is shortly before 5 weeks, and by 6 weeks a yolk sac is seen. The fetal heart pulsation may be seen at 6 weeks, but more commonly at 7 weeks (Figure 11.19, on DVD). At this stage in pregnancy, there is no individual variation and a normal pregnancy grows at a predictable rate. By 7 weeks gestation the fetal pole measures 10 mm in length. The fetal length or crown–rump length relates precisely to gestation until 13 weeks. Thereafter head measurement, either bi-parietal diameter (BPD) or head circumference (HC), is appropriate. Early recognition of multiple gestations is important.

The crown–rump measurement is performed with the fetus in profile in a neutral position, measuring the greatest distance from the head to rump, and excluding the legs (Figure 11.20, on DVD). Beyond 13 weeks, the degree of flexion or extension of the fetus makes the measurement unreliable. The period before 13 weeks is one of rapid predictable growth, and fetal length gives accurate dating.

Dating beyond 10–11 weeks will incidentally give additional information. This includes the presence of a normally formed head; identification of the stomach, bladder, four limbs, abdominal cord insertion, placental site and liquor volume. Anomalies identified at this stage are uncommon, but they are significant when they are seen, e.g. anencephaly. Cystic hygroma, an anomaly of lymphatic drainage with an incidence about 3 per 1000 pregnancies (Figures 11.21, 11.22, 11.23 and 11.24, all on DVD), has a high association with chromosome anomaly, typically Turner's syndrome 45X0 (70%), but also Trisomy 18 and 21, and is linked with congenital heart disease. Megacystis, also diagnosable at this gestation, a rare obstructive disorder of the bladder associated with renal dysplasia, similarly carries a poor prognosis (Figure 11.25, on DVD).

THE ANOMALY SCAN

An ultrasound scan specifically for fetal anomalies is typically performed at 20 weeks gestation, but is sometimes delayed to 22 weeks if the mother has a high BMI. This gestation is a compromise when as much information can be obtained from a single examination. It comprises biometric measurements and a systematic review of fetal anatomy. The national standard for the minimum content of this examination is defined (RCOG 2000), but will change with more emphasis on cardiac screening.

STANDARD BIOMETRIC MEASUREMENTS

There has been a progressive standardization of ultrasound charts in UK practice and the reader is referred to those published by the British Medical Ultrasound Society (BMUS).

The bi-parietal diameter (BPD) may vary slightly with variation in head shape. The measurement is made by placing one point of the callipers on the leading edge of the near skull bone and the other point on the leading edge of the far skull bone (Figure 11.26, on DVD). Now head circumference (HC) is favored, measured either by applying crossed diameters across the maximum diameters of the head (Figure 11.27) or tracing the outline. The outline is particularly useful when head shape deviates from normal, as with dolichocephaly

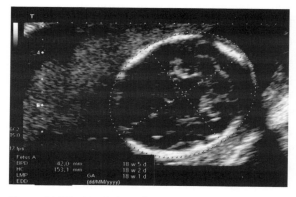

Figure 11.27 Head circumference – use of cross diameters.

(Figure 11.28, on DVD). The correct plane is essential to show a symmetrical shape with a clear view of the ventricles. If the correct plane cannot be obtained by virtue of fetal position, then wait for the fetus to move, or ask the mother to move around to facilitate this position.

The abdominal circumference (AC) is the most variable measurement, and will increase if the fetus is flexed or shows breathing movements. Sometimes several measurements to obtain consistency will improve the accuracy (Figure 11.29, on DVD).

The femur length (FL) is a simple linear measurement, ideally made with the bone orientated across the screen to measure its maximum length.

Review of anatomy

HEAD AND SPINE

Head symmetry is the norm, with a clear midline. The lateral ventricles show symmetry with the choroid plexus within. The maximum width of each lateral ventricle should not exceed 10 mm. The ventricles can be visualized at 12 weeks on the dating scan (Figure 11.30, on DVD) and with equal clarity at 20 weeks (Figure 11.31, on DVD). The cerebellum in the posterior fossa is dumb-bell shaped and its transverse diameter in millimeters is closely equivalent to gestational age in weeks (Figure 11.32, on DVD). Deviation in shape of the cerebellum, classically the banana shape, is indicative of a neural tube defect even when none can be visualized. In more gross examples, the head is characterized as lemon-shaped (Figure 11.33, on DVD).

The fetal spine has a primary curve, which shows as a gentle "C" shape from neck to sacrum. The sacrum reaches a blunted point. When scanning down the spine in either transverse or longitudinal section, continuity is the norm and a break in the pattern requires closer scrutiny (Figure 11.34). Check the skin covering for either a gap or a cystic swelling. Any acute angulation of the spine may be due to a hemi-vertebra.

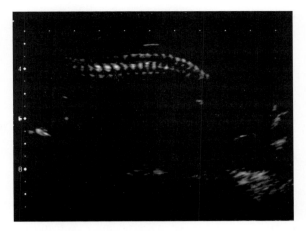

Figure 11.34 Normal fetal spine.

CHEST

View the thorax and abdomen in profile and transversely; the stomach is always below the heart and on the left. The diaphragm is seen as a faint line in profile and will move periodically. Scanning down transversely through the lung fields shows an even texture either side of the heart. The presence of bowel or stomach within the chest is indicative of diaphragmatic hernia. The diameter of the normal heart is never more than half the thoracic diameter and the heart occupies about one third of the thorax.

FETAL HEART

The basic four-chamber view of the fetal heart will exclude more than 90% of all major cardiac anomalies. The importance in screening is to ensure that this view is obtained consistently. The ideal position is for the fetus to face the probe and visualize the chambers via the anterior chest wall. If the fetus rotates away, shadowing from the spine causes significant signal drop-out, and if it will not move, the examination may have to be repeated. The required view is a horizontal section through the thorax just above the diaphragm, which includes a rib to ensure the section is truly transverse. The orientation of the heart is that the left atrium lies closest to the descending aorta (Figures 11.35 and 11.36, both on DVD).

When the anatomy is abnormal, the relationship between the left atrium and the aorta remains fairly constant. The four-chamber view shows the following features.

- The ventricles are equal in size and move synchronously, the atria likewise.
- There is continuity along the ventricular septum, which may be better seen by rotating the probe so that the septum lies across the axis of the ultrasound beam.
- The crus or central cross is offset and always present. The atrial septum is open in fetal life but is guarded by a valve flap, which may be seen with heart movement.

If any anomaly appears to be present, remember the constant relationship of the left atrium to the aorta and check the stomach is on the left.

ABDOMEN

The stomach lies on the left under the diaphragm and is well delineated being fluid-filled (Figure 11.37, on DVD). Its absence on scan is unusual and warrants a second look.

The bladder is abdominal in the fetus since the bony pelvis is shallow. Failure to see it may indicate recent emptying, and a second look is useful. A functional bladder implies normal renal function. The kidneys appear relatively large in the fetus either side of the spine beneath the diaphragm. Dilatation of the renal pelvis is not uncommon, 5 mm or less being normal.

Bowel gives an amorphous reflection at 20 weeks. Only in late pregnancy can normal colon be distinguished. Hyperechoic bowel may be indicative of pathology. To meet the diagnostic criteria for "echogenic bowel", the gain must be turned down and the bowel reflections need to be at least as bright as bone. The associated pathologies to be considered are swallowed blood, intra-uterine infection

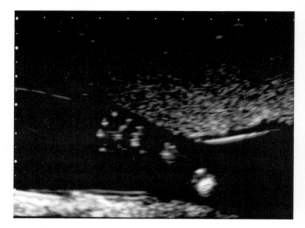

Figure 11.40   Fetal hand at 12 weeks.

and cystic fibrosis. This "soft marker" can trigger other appropriate investigations.

The cord insertion is placed in the midline and is a perpendicular to the abdominal wall (Figure 11.38, on DVD). If the cord emerges from a sac at this point, then the lesion is an exomphalus, whereas if free loops of bowel lie outside of the abdominal wall the lesion is a gastroschisis (Figure 11.39, on DVD). Exomphalus is associated with Trisomy in 30% of fetuses and is an indication for karyotyping.

LIMBS

Each limb contains three long bones, the visualization of which is indicative of the integrity of the limb. Hands and feet are not as clearly seen. The hand can often be seen outstretched at 12 weeks (Figure 11.40). It is more likely to be in a neutral position at 20 weeks (Figure 11.41, on DVD), and often the scan does not give a clear image of the fingers. At times only more prolonged observation of hand movements will provide this view. The feet are naturally flat and require a profile view. Both hands and both feet must be seen to confirm normality (Figure 11.42, on DVD). The absence of a hand or deformity is apparent by the time of the standard anomaly scan at 20 weeks (Figures 11.43a and 11.43b, both on DVD).

FACE AND LIPS

Cleft lip, defects of the alveolar ridge and palate are eminently correctable but initially quite striking when at birth we relate so much to the baby's face. Early identification and counseling by a dedicated regional team can lessen this impact. A facial profile is useful (Figure 11.44, on DVD), but more correctly a coronal view of nose and lips will exclude a defect (Figure 11.45, on DVD). However, if the fetus persistently faces away from the examining probe this view may not be attained.

THE PLACENTA AND CORD

The position of the placenta is a function of the area available and is usually anterior, posterior or fundal. Many placentae are low on early scans and are only significant if they completely cover the cervical os at 20 weeks. The texture is uniform and speckled in early pregnancy, becoming more patterned as pregnancy progresses due to calcification. Occasional cysts and vascular lakes are usually of no significance and diminish as the placenta grows. Placental shape is variable, as is the point of cord insertion. Generally a placenta, which reaches the fundus, will never amount to placenta previa (Figure 11.46). An unusual placental shape is illustrated where a significant thickness of placenta was present

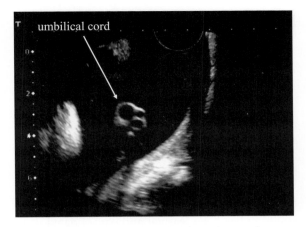

Figure 11.49a   Transverse section through normal 3-vessel umbilical cord.

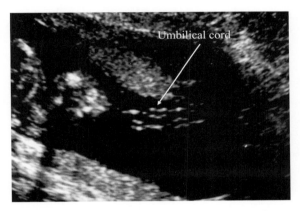

Figure 11.49b   Normal 3-vessel cord along its length.

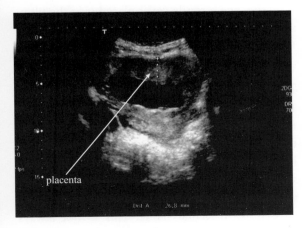

Figure 11.46   Placenta previa.

high on the posterior wall reaching the fundus, yet a lobe extending sufficiently low to create previa with placental tissue encircling the lower uterine segment (Figure 11.47, on DVD). On rare occasions late in pregnancy, TVS imaging of the cervix and lower placenta will provide certainty about placental position, particularly when the shadowing of a well-calcified fetal head hides the lower segment wall (Figure 11.48, on DVD).

A normal cord contains two arteries and one vein (Figures 11.49a and 11.49b). The two-vessel cord, one artery and one vein, may be associated with unilateral renal agenesis, and it is worth rechecking this.

Table 11.1 Indications for amniocentesis

- Fetal karyotyping
- Liquor examination for viruses by PCR and culture
- Fetal blood grouping
- Biochemical testing for inherited disorders of metabolism
- Fetal sexing for X-linked disorders

Table 11.2 Informed consent for amniocentesis

Main considerations

- Miscarriage rate of 1%
- Failed culture rate of approximately 1 in 300
- Maternal cell contamination
- Unclear results from cultures occasionally due to mosaicism
- Unexpected results
- Printed information sheet and written consent

Table 11.3 Equipment for amniocentesis

- 20 ml syringe
- Amniocentesis needle (length 120 mm)
- Sterile towels or paper
- Sterile bag, sheath for transducer
- Sterile ultrasound gel
- Chlorhexidine lotion or spray

Amniocentesis

This technique of ultrasound-directed sampling of amniotic fluid is one to perform once other basic scanning has been learned and consolidated. It is described in detail since the technique is relevant to other situations. It is the commonest diagnostic test performed in pregnancy and is offered to about 5% of pregnant women (Table 11.1). A starting point for training is the ultrasound phantom, the importance being to learn to direct the amniocentesis needle within the plane of the ultrasound beam along its entire length and visualize it continuously while it remains within the uterus, so keeping the risk of fetal trauma to a minimum.

The procedure

The procedure can be performed from 15 weeks onwards. The author uses local anesthetic, but it is not essential. It has the advantage that provided the needle path has been anesthetized the patient will be able to keep still if the intended target is small.

Informed consent

Written, informed consent prior to the procedure is recommended, which should include giving an information leaflet, with either local or national statistics and complications (Table 11.2) (RCOG green top guideline on amniocentesis).

Preparation for amniocentesis

The layout is described for a right-handed operator. The couch is adjusted to the appropriate height. The operator sits on the patient's left at right angles, facing the scanner screen on the opposite side. The trolley with the needles, syringes and towels is immediately to the side of the operator's right hand for economy of movement (Table 11.3).

The maternal abdomen is exposed as for a clinical examination, and cleansed with antiseptic, usually chlorhexidine. Aseptic technique is used throughout. The abdomen is draped, exposing the procedure site, and a sterile cover placed over the ultrasound transducer into which gel has been placed to facilitate sound conductivity.

Technique

The needle may be inserted via a needle guide mounted on the transducer itself or a free-hand technique, which is favored by the author. A preliminary scan is used to confirm the pregnancy is a singleton and viable, then identify a liquor pool, which ideally contains no fetal parts and is not crossed by placental tissue. This is not always possible.

Table 11.4 Post-test advice

Return with symptoms of concern
- Persistently unwell
- Pyrexia of 38 °C
- Fluid loss vaginally
- Pain unrelieved by paracetamol
- Vaginal bleeding
- Abdominal pain

The liquor pool is visualized holding the transducer still in the left hand, allowing space for needle access from the side of the transducer. If local anesthetic is used, place it from skin down to peritoneum and use the needle as a guide for the subsequent angle of approach for the amniocentesis needle. Keep the transducer still. Place the amniocentesis needle with a series of short stabbing motions directed in the plane of the transducer beam. The needle approaches the target pool by passing underneath the transducer and is visualized along its entire length (Figure 11.50, on DVD).

The scan shows entry with no placental tissue or fetal part in the sampling field. Where there is no suitable window, transplacental entry is performed (Figure 11.51, on DVD), keeping to the placental edge or the thinnest portion as much as possible. The deepest available pool may not always lie in an anatomical plane. The incidence of fetal loss does not appear to be increased. The transducer must be kept stationary at all times whichever method is used, and only the needle moved. Once the needle is placed in the liquor, fluid can be drawn off free-hand, using a syringe holder, or by an assistant. On completion, when withdrawing the needle anticipate a transient stream of bleeding from the fetal surface of the placenta, which is self-limiting. Confirm the presence of the fetal heart after the procedure. If the mother is Rhesus-negative, the procedure is covered with 250 IU of anti-D when performed below 20 weeks gestation (Table 11.4).

Avoiding problems at amniocentesis

Always reduce distractions in the room, and ensure the patient is comfortable and able to lie still. Abdominal muscle movement can deflect the needle off course. Avoid passing the needle close to the umbilicus: it is both sensitive and the tissues are tougher. The deepest accessible pool may lie in any plane, not always the long axis. Ensure no bowel lies between the abdominal wall and the uterus by applying steady pressure with the transducer. A posterior placenta always displaces the fetus forwards, closer to the amniocentesis needle. In this situation, avoid over-passing the needle, as this may traumatize the placenta and cause bloodstaining of the liquor specimen. This can be avoided by approaching laterally, which may give more space.

If at any point the needle tip cannot be seen, then stop, leave the needle in position and move the transducer until it can be seen. If the travel is off course, then partly withdraw, recheck position and continue. If the needle entry through the uterine wall is too gentle the amnion may "tent": a sharp tap or stab should pierce this. Check there is sufficient room to allow the additional travel of the needle.

Cytogenetic analysis may fail when a liquor specimen is blood-stained. If on aspiration there is blood-staining from entry through the uterine wall, then discard the initial liquor and use a new syringe.

Results

The type of service provided by the regional laboratories varies slightly. Rapid testing by QF-PCR for limited conditions, e.g. trisomy 13, 18, 21, may be available within 3 working days, whereas full amniocyte culture takes about 2.5 weeks. Ongoing audit of this practice is the best way to assess complication rates and competency.

FURTHER READING

Routine Ultrasound Screening in Pregnancy. Protocols, Standards and Training. Report of the RCOG Working Party. RCOG Press. July 2000. ISBN 1 900364 43 3.

Intimate Examinations. Report of a Working Party. Section 5.4 RCOG Press. September 1997. ISBN 1 900364 06 9.

www.gestation.net: Customised growth charts and birthweight centiles.

www.bmus.org. Ultrasound safety. British Medical Ultrasound Society (BMUS).

www.screeningservices.org.uk/asw: Antenatal Screening Wales.

www.arc-uk.org: Antenatal results and choices.

www.fetalmedicine.com: Nuchal translucency screening (Downs screening 11–13 weeks).

www.rcog.org.uk: Greentop guideline on amniocentesis.

Chapter 12

Ultrasound in ophthalmic anesthesia

CHANDRA M. KUMAR

Introduction

The benefits of directly visualizing targeted nerve structures and monitoring the distribution of local anesthetic are significant [1]. Direct visualization improves the quality of nerve blocks and avoids complications [2]. The relevant anatomy can be demonstrated and many structures that regional anesthetists seek to avoid are clearly shown [1]. Ultrasound imaging also plays an important and enduring part of the training of regional anesthetists.

The application of ultrasound in the field of ophthalmology has steadily increased over time due to the availability of superior instruments and improvement in examination techniques [3]. Ultrasound is used to measure the parts of the eye, document pathology, and examine inside the eye. This now constitutes a nearly ideal examining modality for the eye and is an essential tool of the trade. Although ultrasound modality has limited applications in the field of ophthalmic anesthesia, they are likely to increase. Therefore, it is important to understand the basic principles of physics relevant to ultrasound. The readers are advised to read chapters devoted to physics in this book and other textbooks on ultrasound [4–7]. This chapter contains the essential physics of ultrasound relevant to the eye, how to perform an ultrasound in clinical practice, and its application in ophthalmic anesthesia.

Basic physics

Ultrasound utilizes sound waves to form an image of the eye. High-frequency sound waves are emitted from a probe. The sound waves travel through the eye and reflect from ocular structures back to the emitter probe. The probe receives the sound waves and converts them into the image that appears on the examiner's screen as an ultrasound echo.

Ultrasound is an acoustic wave that is not visible. Waves consist of an oscillation of particles within a medium. Waves which have frequencies greater than 20 kHz (20 000 oscillations/s) are inaudible to humans. For the best imaging of the orbit, 8–10 MHz (millions of cycles per second) is used for general orbital structures but a frequency of 50–60 MHz is used for the anterior segment of the eye. Very high frequencies produce short wavelengths which allow resolution of minute ocular and orbital structures. Ultrasound is propagated as a longitudinal wave that consists of alternating compressions and refractions of molecules as the waves pass through a medium. Liquid medium such as aqueous and vitreous are very compressible and sound waves travel slowly. Solid media are less compressible, hence waves are transmitted faster. As

Ultrasound in Anesthetic Practice, ed. Graham Arthurs and Barry Nicholls. Published by Cambridge University Press.
© Cambridge University Press 2009.

longitudinal waves travel through the tissue, part of the wave may be reflected back towards the transducer (source of the emitted energy) and this reflected wave is referred to as an echo (graphic presentation of sound echoes). Returning echoes may be affected by many factors such as absorption, refraction, angle of sound incidence, size, shape and smoothness of acoustic interfaces.

The piezo-electric effect of certain thin crystal and ceramic materials is used. This effect is characterized by the emission of a specific sound wavelength through the deformation of the crystal when it is stimulated by an alternating electrical potential. Conversely, the crystal can receive echoes of the same wavelength and convert them into electrical potentials. This alternating emission–reception arrangement is known as the pulse–echo system of ultrasound. The resonating crystal or ceramic with its dampening, focusing and electrical circuits are incorporated into the transducer. High-frequency sound waves are emitted from a single probe that contains both the transmitter and receiver, towards the target tissues. Various structures in its path will reflect separate echoes back towards the probe arriving at different times. Those reflected from the most distal structures arrive last, having traveled the farthest. As the sound waves bounce back off the various tissue components, they are detected by the transducer.

There are different types of probes. The probe is placed in contact with the skin with the eyelids closed. These probes produce poor views of the anterior chamber of the eye. If it is essential to image any area in detail in the absence of a higher-frequency transducer, an open waterbath scan or an immersion technique with the probe in direct contact with the globe is required. As access to the orbit is limited, scanning is done in both longitudinal and transverse planes with the patients looking straight, up, down, left and right. Posterior compartment abnormalities are observed in real time during rapid eye movements. Recent advances in instrument design and specification have resulted in the production of high-quality, ophthalmic-dedicated ultrasound equipment incorporating different types of probes, real-time kinetic properties with high-resolution images.

Ultrasound echoes received by the probe are amplified and signals are presented on the oscilloscope. A time–amplitude trace depicts the echoes as spikes with the vertical axis relating to the strength of reflectance properties, whereas the time scale on the horizontal axis indirectly depicts a distance scale. These can be displayed in several images formats.

A-scan (amplitude mode)

This format is based on conversion of time elapsed between echoes and the known speed of sound in the medium. The A-scan is a one-dimensional display of sound waves. The sound beam is aimed in a straight line. Each time a sound wave hits a structure in the eye, a spike is formed on the screen whose amplitude is dependent on the density of the reflecting tissue (Figures 12.1 and 12.2, both on DVD). The height and spacing between each of the echoes provides the examiner with valuable information. The spikes are arranged in temporal sequence, with the latency of each signal's arrival correlating with that structure's distance from the probe. Temporal separation can be used to calculate the distance between the points, based on the speed of sound in that tissue medium. A-scans are most commonly used to measure the axial length and determine the appropriate intraocular lens for cataract surgery.

B-scan (brightness mode)

If an A-scan probe is swept across the eye, a continuous series of individual A-scans is obtained. From spatial summation of these multiple linear scans, a two-dimensional cross-sectional view of the eye is constructed. Echoes are presented as dots rather than spikes. The position of the echo is therefore the same as on an A-scan, but the intensity of the dots relates to the intensity of reflection. Therefore a B-scan image is composed of innumerable echo dots that are integrated from different beam locations as the transducer sweeps across the object in one plane (Figures 12.3 and 12.4, both on DVD). The resulting graphic two-dimensional image depicts outlines and internal tissue echoes of the object, resembling a thin histological section. This scan is extremely valuable when the view inside the eye is obstructed by blood, dense cataract, or other cloudy media.

Doppler ultrasound

The Doppler effect describes the effects of motion on the reflected frequency of waves. An object moving towards a point will reflect back signals at a higher frequency, and vice versa. The amount of change in the frequency (Doppler shift) is proportional to the speed of the object, and so a measurement of flow can be made by a mathematical formula. The major reflectors are blood cells. The electronics allow the detection of the difference between normal reflections and reflections that have undergone Doppler shift. Doppler signals are documented as auditory changes in frequency, or they are shown on a strip graph chart. There are several different ways in which the Doppler image can be depicted. Color Doppler gives an estimate of flow rate and represents it as a color against a gray background (red towards, blue away). The color display represents direction of flow. Pulsed Doppler allows a sample to be taken by a quick pulse of sound, allowing a graphic representation of flow. Power Doppler shows the power of the Doppler signal as opposed to the amount of Doppler shift.

Examination technique

For vitreo-retinal assessment, B-scan ultrasonography is commonly used. Anesthetists are more likely to deal with this mode of scan. Examination technique can only be perfected by training and practice.

The type of examination performed is determined by the indication for examination. The patient is seated in a reclinable chair of adjustable height. An ultrasound machine is also placed on an examining table of adjustable height. The patient's head and the instrument are situated close together, so that the probe position and the screen may be viewed simultaneously. Topical anesthesia is applied to the eye before the examination if the probe is likely to be applied directly to the globe.

It is important that the examiner must have the ability to think three-dimensionally while examining the globe with instruments that only have one- or two-dimensional displays. The ultrasound probe is clearly annotated to indicate the direction of scanning and its orientation with respect to the display on the monitor. Each probe has a marker, usually a dot, line or logo that indicates the side of the probe that is represented on the upper portion of the display screen. The probe face is always represented by the initial line that appears on the left side of the echogram. The right side of the echogram indicates the region of the eye located opposite the probe face. The upper part of the echogram corresponds to the portion of the globe where the probe marker is directed. The center of the screen corresponds to the central portion of the probe face.

Methylcellulose gel is applied to the face of the B-scan probe as a coupling medium. The patient should be asked to look down with the eye opened and the probe should be applied to the upper lid. The upper part of the fundus is examined through the lower lid and with the eye looking up. The probe is placed in horizontal, vertical and oblique orientation. Horizontal scans are usually taken to build up a three-dimensional image. Additional vertical and oblique scans may give extra information. Although modern scanners have good lateral resolution, the best image is acquired with the center of the beam. If the area of interest is upper nasal quadrant, the patient is asked to look up and nasally.

In a horizontal scan, the probe is placed on the globe so that back-and-forth movements of the transducer occur parallel (tangential) to the limbus.

This causes the sound beam to move back and forth across the opposite fundus, producing a circumferential slice through several meridians of globe. By convention, horizontal transverse scans (12 or 6 o'clock meridians) are performed with the marker oriented towards the patient's nose. Therefore, the upper part of the echogram always represents the nasal portion of the globe. On the other hand, vertical transverse scans (3 or 9 o'clock meridians) are performed with the marker directed superiorly so the top of the echogram represents the upper portion of the globe. In oblique transverse scans, the probe is place at half past the hour clock marks.

In a vertical scan, the probe face is rotated 90° from the position used for the transverse scan. This means that the back-and-forth movement of the transducer is oriented perpendicular to the limbus.

In an oblique scan, the patient fixates the eye in primary gaze and the probe is placed on the center of the globe, thereby displaying the lens and the optic nerve in the center of the echogram. The optic nerve is used as an anatomic reference for the posterior fundus.

The ultrasound probe is applied in a systematic fashion and usually there is a protocol which every examiner must follow because ultrasonography is a dynamic form of clinical examination. The echoes on the oscilloscope are constantly changing to reflect changes in probe position, transducer frequency and receiver sensitivity. Kinetic information obtained during the course of the examination should be documented by using a video recorder if a real-time system is compatible with the recorder. Photographs are usually taken of the oscilloscope screen for documentation of findings.

Uses of ultrasound in ophthalmic anesthesia

Ultrasound is considered an essential tool in the investigation and management of many ophthalmic diseases. Ultrasound is used to examine, diagnose and assess the morbidity related to needle or cannula damage during ophthalmic regional anesthesia which is known to occur [8]. A prompt diagnosis and early management can reduce the ill effects of these complications. It is therefore important to be familiar with normal and abnormal images which may be encountered in anesthetic practice.

Clinical use of the A-scan
Axial length measurement

Measurement of the axial length of the globe is usually performed in patients scheduled for cataract surgery to calculate the replacement power of the lens. Knowledge of the axial length measurement is an essential prerequisite before embarking on a needle block, as the incidence of predicted perforation rate increases when a needle block is performed in patients whose axial length is greater than 26 mm [9]. Early diagnosis and treatment are known to save a majority of damaged eyes [9, 10].

Clinical uses of the B-scan

In the normal orbit, a transverse or equatorial B-scan demonstrates an anatomical cross-section with readily recognizable anatomical structures. The anterior and posterior surfaces of the lens produce strong echoes where they are at right angles to the beam, and the ciliary apparatus by the side of the lens also gives rise to strong echoes. The aqueous and vitreous chambers are completely free of echoes. The outline of the retinal surface is smooth, but a small dimple is sometimes seen at the insertion of the optic nerve, and a small apparent elevation in the midline of the globe posteriorly due to slightly higher velocity of sound through the lens. The optic nerve (Figure 12.5, on DVD) can be seen as an ill-defined echo, a linear structure passing through the highly refractive retro-orbital fat. Retrobulbar fat is readily identified as strong echoes. Medial and lateral rectus muscles can be

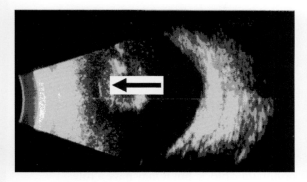

Figure 12.6 Cataractous lens.

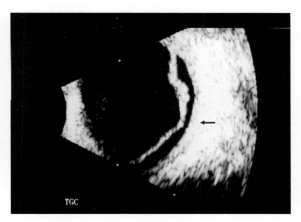

Figure 12.8 Retinal detachment.

identified as spindle-shaped, echo-poor structures, 4 mm in thickness.

Cataract

Ultrasound of the eye is performed to confirm the normality of the vitreous chamber and to exclude pathology such as retinal detachment or choroidal melanoma before cataract surgery. The lens is not very echogenic if there is no cataract. The mature cataractous lens produces low-level echoes which are often difficult to demonstrate, but at the earlier hydropic stage the lamellation of the lens becomes apparent as it swells due to the absorption of fluid. A thick rim of increased echogenicity is seen when the cataract is very dense (Figure 12.6).

Retinal detachment

Detachment of the retina can occur following orbital block, particularly following perforation of the globe during injection or secondary to severe retrobulbar hemorrhage [8]. Detachment gives rise to linear structures lying within the vitreous attached to the optic nerve insertion. The detached retina is usually mobile and can be see to exhibit wave-like movements when the position of the eye is changed rapidly (Figures 12.7, on DVD, 12.8 and 12.9, on DVD). The ultrasonic features are usually distinctive, the detached retina forming a V- or Y-shaped arrangement of echoes extending from the ora serata to the optic nerve head, where it is

tethered by the optic nerve filaments. It is important to differentiate this from vitreous membrane that may occur in patients with chronic vitreous hemorrhage, but these are not attached to the optic nerve.

Vitreous hemorrhage

Vitreous hemorrhage is a rare complication of orbital block. Hemorrhage into the vitreous gives rise to detectable low-level echoes which coalesce to form linear or focal structures throughout the vitreous (Figure 12.10, on DVD). A large hemorrhage appears as irregular hyperechoic areas within the anechoic vitreous. Small hemorrhages may be difficult to demonstrate.

Orbital cellulitis

Recently, many cases of explained and unexplained orbital cellulitis have been reported [11, 12]. Ultrasound is one of the essential tools in the diagnosis, assessment and monitoring the process of recovery in these cases. Inflammation and congestion of orbital structures sometimes may not show changes and produces a normal ultrasonic pattern [4]. Inflammatory ultrasound findings may be diffuse, or localized to a particular area or tissue. Inflammatory changes are clearly distinguished from the findings associated with

173

neoplasm. Cellulitis and pseudotumor (idiopathic orbital inflammation) produce diffuse orbital ultrasound findings. The retrobulbar fat is generally the most involved tissue, with an abnormally diffuse mottled texture identified ultrasonically by widening of the spaces between echoes. These changes probably result from interstitial edema separating fat globules and connective tissue abnormalities [4].

Trauma

Perforation or penetration of the globe, although rare, can be a sight-threatening situation after orbital block. Penetrating eye injury should be investigated with caution. Perforation of the globe can lead to loss of aqueous fluid, reduction in the size of the anterior chamber and diminution of globe volume following vitreous loss, and this can be seen by reduced axial length. The presence of hemorrhage and intraocular foreign bodies are well seen and can be located accurately. Ultrasound can also differentiate between intraocular and extraocular foreign bodies, and help in their surgical removal. In patients with recent injury or who have undergone recent cataract surgery, a trapped air bubble may be interpreted as a foreign body.

Other uses of B-scan ultrasound in ophthalmic anesthesia
Placement of needles and catheters

Retrobulbar and peribulbar injections are performed to deliver local anesthetic agent and other medications. These injections are performed without guidance and can lead to complications that are rare but visually devastating when they occur. The needle may penetrate the optic nerve, perforate the globe and disperse toxic quantities of drugs intraocularly. Ultrasound can help to locate the needle tip entering the intraconal area during retrobulbar block [13, 14] but others [15] have reported difficulty in locating the tip of a retrobulbar and peribulbar needle. Prolonged anesthesia using a catheter

for ophthalmic block has been described. It is possible for a catheter that is inserted through the needle to end up in an unusual position. Ultrasound-guided placement of indwelling catheters in both peribulbar and retrobulbar spaces has been used for prolonged anesthesia as well as for post-operative pain relief [16]. At present there is not enough evidence to recommend the routine use of ultrasound in the placement of a needle or a catheter during ophthalmic block, but it may have a role.

Localization of anesthetic fluid during injection

Injection of local anesthetic agent around the orbit by needle or cannula usually leads to anesthesia, but the mechanism is not very well understood. The passage of local anesthetic following peribulbar, retrobulbar and sub-Tenon's block has now been extensively studied [15, 17]. The spread of injected local anesthetic agent during retrobulbar block is less easily identifiable, but fluid can be seen to be localized within the cone and distributed in the intraconal fat. The identification of peribulbar fluid is similarly difficult, but the fluid is seen in the extraconal fat. The situation is much better understood during sub-Tenon's block. Anesthetic fluid is easily seen distributed around the globe during sub-Tenon's block (Figure 12.11). The fluid around the optic nerve develops a characteristics T-sign [15, 17].

Measurement of ocular blood flow

Ocular blood flow is significantly impaired during regional orbital anesthesia [18–25]. Color Doppler ultrasound is capable of measuring small fluctuations in ocular blood flow. Blood flow in the central retinal artery, posterior ciliary arteries, ophthalmic artery and central retinal vein can be measured. Measurement of ocular blood flow may be crucial in patients whose ocular circulation is compromised where regional ophthalmic anesthesia is being used [24–26].

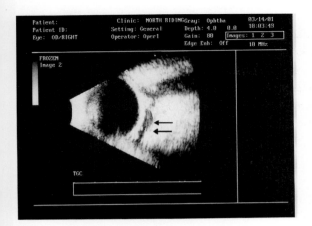

Figure 12.11 T-sign during sub-Tenon injection.

Evaluation of regional ophthalmic techniques

Sub-Tenon's block is performed by introducing a cannula below the Tenon capsule. A variety of cannulae of varying lengths and sizes are available [27]. Even a very small sub-Tenon's cannula is capable of producing anesthesia and akinesia, but evidence to prove how it works is very valuable. A recent study confirms that anesthetic agent is capable of entering the sub-Tenon's space using an ultrashort sub-Tenon cannula giving a characteristic T-sign [28].

Newer developments
Ultrasound biomicroscopy (UBM)

The majority of clinical ultrasound devices operate at a frequency between 1 and 10 MHz, but poly vinylidene difluoride (PVDF) transducers are capable of generating high-frequency ultrasound in the range of 20–100 MHz. These have low mechanical impedance and broad band properties. It has proved to be very valuable owing to a very high frequency. There is no report of the use of this modality in ophthalmic anesthesia.

Power Doppler

Power Doppler is a new modification of Doppler ultrasound that displays the strength of Doppler signal, in addition to the velocity and directional information normally obtained from color Doppler. Power Doppler has three times the sensitivity of conventional ultrasound in detecting blood flow. It is also capable of visualizing much smaller vascular architecture. Doppler is specifically useful in imaging blood flow and vascular lesions of the globe and orbit. At present this equipment has not been used in ophthalmic anesthesia.

Other promising developments in ultrasound in general include three-dimensional imaging, refinement in transducer material and technology leading to improvement in sensitivity and bandwidth.

Ultra-fast B-probe with integrated 3D scanning

The new patented magnetic-driven B-probe design allows an unprecedented scanning rate of B-scan at 50 frames per second for exquisite dynamic motion resolution, and super-fast 3D scanning. The 12 MHz operating frequency offers significantly improved resolution. The 115 dB dynamic range allows gain and contrast to be adjusted during and/or after a scan has been captured, with no loss of information. A scanning rate of 50 frames/s provides excellent motion capture, supported by the industry's most advanced dynamic capture, review and editing capabilities before the movie is stored in the patient database. The 3D rotation motor is integrated inside the B-probe, making 3D scanning far easier than ever before. The integrated 3D B-probe eliminates the need to interrupt the B-scan exam to prepare for 3D scanning. The user just presses the foot switch to obtain a 3D scan in less than 2 s. The two-second scan capture time eliminates most motion artifacts and makes 3D practical even for difficult patients.

Summary

Ultrasonography is a rapid, non-invasive modality that provides detailed examination and resolution of the intraocular structures and soft

175

tissues surrounding the orbit. At present, the application of ultrasound is limited in the field of ophthalmic anesthesia, but its use is likely to increase as more evidence emerges, while ultrasound enthusiasts continue to claim that its use will produce faster, safer and more successful blocks.

REFERENCES

1. Denny NM, Harrop-Griffiths W. 2005. Location, location, location! Ultrasound imaging in regional anaesthesia. *British Journal of Anaesthesia* 2005;94:1–3.

2. Marhofer P, Greher M, Kapral S. Ultrasound guidance in regional anaesthesia. *British Journal of Anaesthesia* 2005;94:7–17.

3. Atta HR. 1999. New applications in ultrasound technology. *British Journal of Ophthalmology* 1999;83:1246–9.

4. Albert DM, Jakobiec FA. 1993. *Principles and Practice of Ophthalmology.* Volume 5. Philadelphia: W.B. Saunders, 1993.

5. Atta HR. *Ophthalmic Ultrasound: A Practical Guide.* London: Churchill Livingstone, 1996.

6. Taylor RH, Shah P, Murray PI, Burdon A. *Key Topics in Ophthalmology.* 2nd ed. Oxford and New York, BIOS Scientific Publishers, 2001.

7. Byrne SF, Green RL. *Ultrasound of the Eye and Orbit.* 2nd ed. Philadelphia: Mosby, 2002.

8. Kumar CM, Dodds C, Fanning G. *Ophthalmic Anaesthesia.* The Netherlands: Swets and Zeitlinger, 2002.

9. Duker JS, Belmont JB, Benson WE, et al. Inadvertent globe perforation during retrobulbar and peribulbar anesthesia. Patient characteristics, surgical management, and visual outcome. *Ophthalmology* 1991;98:519–26.

10. Puri P, Verma D, McKibbin M. 1999. Management of ocular perforations resulting from peribulbar anaesthesia. *Indian Journal of Ophthalmology* 1999;47:181–311.

11. Kumar CM, Dowd TC, Dodds C, Boyce R. Orbital swelling following peribulbar and sub-Tenon's anaesthesia. *Eye* 2004;18:418–20.

12. Muqit MM, Saidkasimova S, Gavin M. Acute orbital cellulitis after sub-Tenon's eye block. *Anaesthesia* 2004;59:411–3.

13. Birch AA, Evans M, Redembo E. The ultrasonic localization of retrobulbar needles during retrobulbar block. *Ophthalmology* 1995;102:824–6.

14. Chang BY, Hee WC, Ling R, Broadway DC, Beigi B. Local anaesthetic techniques and pulsatile ocular blood flow. *British Journal of Ophthalmology* 2000;84:1260–3.

15. Winder S, Walker SB, Atta HR. Ultrasonic localization of anesthetic fluid in sub-Tenon's, peribulbar, and retrobulbar techniques. *Journal of Cataract and Refractive Surgery* 1999; 25:56–9.

16. Gombos K, Laszlo CJ, Hatvani I, Vimlati L, Salacz G. A catheter technique in ophthalmic regional anaesthesia. Clinical investigations. *Acta Anaesthesiologica Scandinavia* 2000;44:453–6.

17. Kumar CM, McNeela BJ. Ultrasonic localization of anaesthetic fluid using sub-Tenon's cannulae of three different lengths. *Eye* 2003;17:1003–7.

18. Robinson R, White M, McCann P, Magner J, Eustace P. Effect of anaesthesia on intraocular blood flow. *British Journal of Ophthalmology* 1991;75:92–3.

19. Hulbert MF, Yang YC, Pennefather PM, Moore JK. Pulsatile ocular blood flow and intraocular pressure during retrobulbar injection of lignocaine: influence of additives. *Journal of Glaucoma* 1998; 7:413–6.

20. Findl O, Dallinger S, Menapace R, et al. Effects of peribulbar anesthesia on ocular blood flow in patients undergoing cataract surgery.

American Journal of Ophthalmology 1999;127:645–9.

21. Rainer G, Kiss B, Dallinger S, *et al.* Effect of small incision cataract surgery on ocular blood flow in cataract patients. *Journal of Cataract and Refractive Surgery* 1999;25:964–8.

22. Chang WM, Stetten GD, Lobes LA Jr, Shelton DM, Tamburo RJ. Guidance of retrobulbar injection with real-time tomographic reflection. *Journal of Ultrasound Medicine* 2000;21:1131–5.

23. Watkins R, Beigi B, Yates M, Chang B, Linardos E. Intraocular pressure and pulsatile ocular blood flow after retrobulbar and peribulbar anaesthesia. *British Journal of Ophthalmology* 2001;85:796–8.

24. Coupland SG, Deschenes MC, Hamilton RC. Impairment of ocular blood flow during regional orbital anesthesia. *Canadian Journal of Ophthalmology* 2001;36:140–4.

25. Pianka P, Weintraub-Padova H, Lazar M, Geyer O. Effect of sub-Tenon's and peribulbar anesthesia on intraocular pressure and ocular pulse amplitude. *Journal of Cataract and Refractive Surgery* 2001;27:1221–6.

26. Netland PA, Siegner SW, Harris A. Color Doppler ultrasound measurements after topical and retrobulbar epinephrine in primate eyes. *Investigative Ophthalmology and Visual Science* 1997;38:2655–61.

27. Kumar CM, Dodds C, McLure H, Chabria R. A comparison of three sub-Tenon's cannulae. *Eye* 2004;18:1279.

28. McNeela BJ, Kumar CM. Sub-Tenon's block with an ultrashort cannula. *Journal of Cataract and Refractive Surgery* 2004;30:858–62.

Chapter 13

Use of ultrasound in assessing soft tissue injury

GEOFF HIDE

Introduction

Specific issues for ultrasound of soft tissue

Ultrasound of soft tissue structures and disorders requires practitioners to consider a number of issues which may not apply to ultrasound in other areas. These include how the probe is held, probe frequency, the use of facilities such as Doppler and extended field of view, and artifacts specific to musculoskeletal imaging. Although images may be obtained and diagnoses made without optimizing these aspects, practitioners should strive where possible to utilize every advantage of the modality, and hence should be familiar with all of these issues.

"Musculoskeletal grip"

When practicing ultrasound of the abdomen, sonographers press firmly to obtain good contact, frequently indenting the skin by several centimeters (Figure 13.1, on DVD). The near-field and superficial structures are usually irrelevant and generally poorly demonstrated on curvilinear probes of low frequency. Any distortion of superficial tissue secondary to pressure is therefore of little significance. Even when performing ultrasound of vascular structures with a linear array probe, significant pressure may be applied if ultrasound is being used to guide arterial cannulation. It must of course be reduced to avoid compressing venous structures where these

are of relevance. Ultrasound of the musculoskeletal system requires the operator to vary the amount of pressure applied with the probe and, in addition, to make fine adjustments to probe angulation, particularly when interrogating structures such as tendons. Therefore, it is useful to hold the probe such that the sonographer's little, ring and possibly middle fingertips are in direct contact with the patient's skin. These fingers can then be used as a pivot both to adjust pressure and probe direction (Figure 13.2, on DVD). When interrogating superficial soft tissue masses, one feature to observe is whether the mass is compressible when pressure is applied. It is vital in this situation to ensure that prior to consciously increasing pressure, one has not already compressed the lesion to its maximum deformable state. Consciously reducing probe pressure or even ensuring that a layer of ultrasound jelly clearly separates the surface of the probe and the skin (Figure 13.3, on DVD) ensures that the sonographer can make a correct assessment.

When assessing deep soft tissue structures, for example in a thigh muscle injury, increased pressure may be required to assist visualization of deeper areas of tissue. It is still important to consider reducing pressure in order to observe fluid collection which may be otherwise compressed. This allows adequate visualization of the size of a muscle tear.

Ultrasound in Anesthetic Practice, ed. Graham Arthurs and Barry Nicholls. Published by Cambridge University Press.
© Cambridge University Press 2009.

Probe frequency

Most modern ultrasound systems have variable frequency probes. Typical maximum probe frequencies for musculoskeletal ultrasound are in the range of 15–17 MHz, but may be reduced when imaging deeper structures since the higher-frequency sound is more rapidly attenuated. Sonographers should consider adjusting probe frequency in addition to the machine gain in order to optimize image quality (Figure 13.4, on DVD).

Extended field of view

Individual ultrasound images, particularly with linear array probes, often show limited areas of anatomy and can be difficult for others to orientate. Static images fail to demonstrate and exploit the dynamic advantages of ultrasound, and clinicians undoubtedly find images from other modalities such as MRI easier to understand. Most ultrasound systems now offer an extended field of view facility (Figure 13.5, on DVD), which goes some way towards offsetting this disadvantage. Extended field of view imaging can be difficult where the skin surface is curved, and frequently impossible when the patient is unable to remain still.

Doppler

A full discussion of the uses of various Doppler facilities in the evaluation of vascularity and vascular wave forms is not possible in this chapter, and has been adequately covered elsewhere. Nevertheless, it is important to note that power or color Doppler are required for the full evaluation of soft tissue inflammation and soft tissue masses, and pulsed Doppler is necessary to record the nature of a vascular wave form within a mass satisfactorily. Sonographers should be familiar with the use and pitfalls of Doppler and able to make adjustments to the machine settings in order to obtain an accurate reading.

Musculoskeletal ultrasound artifacts

In common with other imaging modalities, ultrasound suffers from a range of artifacts with which the sonographer must be familiar. In musculoskeletal ultrasound, the most important are anisotropy and refractile shadowing.

Anisotropy

Ultrasound forms images from the sound reflected back to the probe, assessing both the intensity of the echo and its depth, the latter by calculation of depth equalling half the distance travelled by the sound pulse, and distance being the product of the time between the emission and collection of the echo. All machines use an estimation for the speed of sound within soft tissue. Echoes received by the probe are only a small proportion of those which occur in soft tissue, many of which are in alternative directions and do not return to the probe for reading (Figure 13.6). Anisotropy refers to the artifactually dark appearance of a structure which is in fact highly reflective of ultrasound due simply to the reflection occurring in a direction other than back towards the probe. Anisotropy is typically observed in the ultrasound of tendons, which are highly reflective structures due to the closely packed parallel collagen bundles which are orientated in a longitudinal direction. When interrogated by an ultrasound beam which is perpendicular to the tendon, strong echoes are reflected directly back to the probe and the ultrasound machine demonstrates a bright structure on screen (Figure 13.7a). When the ultrasound beam intersects the tendon at other angles (Figure 13.7b), sound is once again reflected strongly by the tendon, but the echoes no longer return to the probe and the machine interprets the tendon to be a structure of much lower reflectivity. Anisotropy is observed in tendons both in their long axis and cross section (Figure 13.8). Since tendon disease (tendinopathy) causes a reduction in the reflectivity of a tendon, anisotropy is an

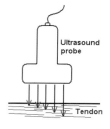

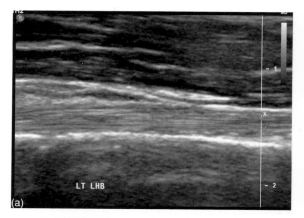

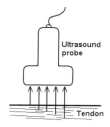

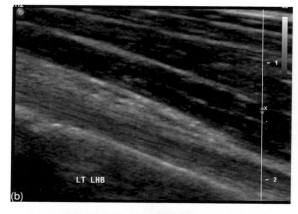

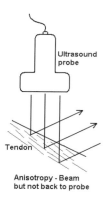

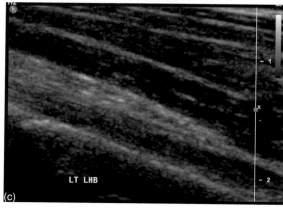

Figure 13.6 Anisotropy.

important mimic of tendon pathology. It is therefore important that sonographers are aware of this artifact and make appropriate adjustments, typically to the probe position in a manner described earlier in this section. Anisotropy can also assist the sonographer to locate a tendon surrounded by other high-reflectivity tissue when scanned in cross section (Figure 13.9, on DVD). In addition to reducing the reflectivity of tendons, tendinopathy also commonly causes tendon swelling, and this is a further important feature to use when

Figure 13.7 Longitudinal US images of the long head of the biceps tendon. Image **a** shows the echogenic tendon insonated at an optimum angle. Note the significant reduction in reflectivity with angulation on image **b** due to anisotropy. This is made even worse on image **c** when compound imaging is turned off. This facility is not available on all US machines.

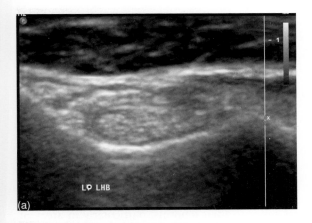

(a)

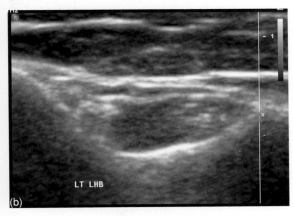

(b)

Figure 13.8 Transverse US images of the long head of the biceps tendon demonstrating anisotropy on image **b** (bottom).

discriminating between anisotropic artifact and true tendon disease.

Refractile shadowing

Refractile shadowing is an artifact which occurs at the edges of reflective structures such as tendons (Figure 13.10, on DVD), where distortion of the sound beam causes shadowing deep to the tendon edge. The appearances are similar to those of posterior acoustic shadowing when the ultrasound beam is totally reflected by a structure such as bone or a gallstone, but the mechanism in this case is refraction of the ultrasound beam rather than reflection. The artifact does obscure detail of

deeper structures, and also makes it difficult to assess changes in reflectivity of the periphery of the tendon, also known as the epitendineum. Refractile shadowing can usually be easily negated by simply moving the probe to a different position such that the area of previously obscured epitendineum is now parallel to the surface of the probe. Refractile shadowing will almost certainly then be observed in areas of previously visualized tendon surface.

Ultrasound anatomy of soft tissue

In order to correctly interpret abnormalities of soft tissue on ultrasound, sonographers must be familiar with the normal appearances of the different tissue and structures which will be encountered. When an ultrasound beam enters a patient, it passes through a series of tissue layers. These are illustrated in Figure 13.11 (on DVD). The ultrasound beam passes initially through the epidermis which is normally only 100 µm thick, although it may be up to 2 mm thick on the palms of the hands and soles of the feet. Next, the beam crosses the dermis, a supporting layer of the skin containing hair follicles, glands and tiny nerves, vessels and lymphatics. The dermis typically measures between 1 and 3 mm thick. Ultrasound cannot distinguish epidermis and dermis separately, and both appear as a uniform, relatively highly reflective layer, normally referred to as skin. Below this, the ultrasound beam traverses the hypodermis, usually referred to as subcutaneous fat. This layer of tissue is much less reflective, but is crossed by thin echogenic septa which appear to be randomly distributed. Further small nerves, vessels and lymphatics are present in this layer, but only the vessels can be identified on ultrasound. The thickness of the hypodermis is extremely variable both in and between individuals. The next layer crossed by the ultrasound beam varies depending on whether the probe is positioned over bone or soft tissue. Bone is covered by a normally thin layer of periosteum which cannot be independently distinguished from the reflective surface of cortical bone in normal cases (Figure 13.12, on DVD). In cases of periosteal thickening or trauma, a distinction can be made. The interface between soft tissue and bone is highly reflective and ultrasound is unable to image beneath the surface of the cortex. Nevertheless, the contour of a bone surface can be well demonstrated allowing the identification of grooves, fossae and bony prominences such as Lister's tubercle on the dorsal aspect of the distal radius, which are highly useful for anatomical localization (Figure 13.13, on DVD).

In areas of soft tissue, the ultrasound beam passes from the hypodermis through a thin, highly reflective layer of deep fascia which separates it from underlying muscle (Figure 13.14, on DVD). The ultrasound appearances of muscle are variable and will be discussed in greater detail. Individual muscle fibers, covered by a network of nerves and capillaries known as endomysium, are grouped into bundles and are of low reflectivity on ultrasound. Muscle bundles are separated from one another by highly reflective fibro-adipose septa, containing further blood vessels and nerves, also known as perimysium, which is seen as a series of parallel highly reflective lines within the muscle tissue (Figure 13.15, on DVD). In cross section, these parallel lines are seen as short lines or dots.

Muscle bundles may be organized in a variety of ways. Bundles grouped parallel to the long axis of the muscle optimize the distance of contraction which can be achieved, and are more commonly encountered in the abdomen, head and neck regions. Bundles with an oblique (pennate) orientation allow greater force over less distance and are more powerful. Both unipennate and bipennate muscle bundle organization is encountered (Figure 13.16, on DVD). Muscles are surrounded by a dense connective tissue layer called the epimysium. Individual muscles are separated from each other by thin layers of fascia and fat. Muscles are attached to bone by tendons which are of variable

lengths, and a fibro-osseous junction also termed an enthesis, a term also used to describe the union of ligament and capsule with bone. A muscle will have at least one, fleshy muscle belly and two tendons, but muscles with multiple bellies and greater than two tendons exist – for example, the rectus femoris, biceps and triceps. The correct identification of individual muscles requires a knowledge of anatomy and is assisted by the use of anatomical atlases and a systematic approach to localization. Muscles can frequently be most easily identified by reference to their tendons, particularly in areas of difficult anatomy such as the forearm and lower leg. Hence when evaluating a muscle injury or tumor, it is frequently important to determine the tendon anatomy at an adjacent joint which can then be traced to the affective muscle.

Muscle blood flow increases dramatically (up to 20-fold) during exercise and this can result in a significant increase in muscle volume. This increase in vascularity can be dramatic when the muscle is examined with Doppler (Figure 13.17, on DVD).

Tendons consist predominantly of parallel, densely packed collagen fiber bundles/fascicles which act as very strong reflectors of ultrasound. As described earlier in this chapter, when the ultrasound beam intersects perpendicular to these fibers, reflection occurs directly back to the probe, and the tendon is interpreted by the machine as a bright structure on the image (Figure 13.18, on DVD). When the beam intersects the tendon at an oblique angle, most of the reflected sound will not be directed back to the probe and therefore the tendon is incorrectly assigned a much darker appearance on the ultrasound image (anisotropy). It is important to note that a tendon forms deep within its muscle belly and gradually thickens as increasing numbers of individual muscle fibers fuse with it along a broad myotendinous junction. Once all muscle fibers have joined the tendon, its cross-sectional area usually remains constant (although its shape may change; for example, if the tendon passes around a bony pulley such as the malleoli at the ankle) until the enthesis is reached. At this point, once again, fibers leave the tendon to fuse with bone and the tendon becomes thinner. The distance over which the tendon thickness changes at the enthesis is usually very much shorter than the myotendinous junction but can be several centimeters in length, particularly at the tibial insertion of the patellar tendon.

Tendons are normally avascular on Doppler. Tendons may be surrounded by either a dense connective tissue layer or a synovial sheath, both of which facilitate tendon movement. The synovial sheath is a cylindrical sack containing a thin film of fluid which serves to lubricate the tendon surface and may be seen as a thin anechoic layer or halo on ultrasound (Figure 13.19, on DVD). Tendons with synovial sheaths are found most commonly in the extremities, particularly at ankle and wrist. Tendons without a synovial sheath are covered by a dense connective tissue layer known as the epitendineum which is highly reflective (Figure 13.20, on DVD). Peripheral to this is a lower reflectivity area of loose connective tissue called the paratenon.

Other structures which are encountered in musculoskeletal ultrasound are joints, bursae, nerves and blood vessels. The latter will not be discussed further (readers are referred to the chapter on vascular ultrasound for a discussion of the appearances of arteries and veins), other than to once again recommend the use of a cross-sectional anatomical atlas as an aid to increasing the knowledge of anatomy.

The appearances of nerves on ultrasound is variable and depends upon the size of the nerve in question, the frequency of ultrasound used, and the angle at which the nerve and the ultrasound beam intersect. Large nerves are typically encountered in close proximity to vessels, and appear as linear hyperechoic structures with a fascicular rather than fibrillar ultrasound pattern (Figure 13.21, on DVD). Nerves are slightly lower in reflectivity than tendons and, although they also show some anisotropy, it is to a less dramatic degree. Modern ultrasound

machines with high-frequency linear probes permit glorious detail of nerve structures to be obtained, and it is possible to follow the terminal branches of the brachial plexus from the axilla to the wrist and the sciatic nerve, and its branches from the ischial spine to the ankle.

Ultrasound of joints and bursae is commonly performed when the structures are inflamed or otherwise distended. It is important to remember that because ultrasound cannot examine deep to cortical bone, a complete evaluation of the articular surfaces of a joint is rarely possible. Nevertheless, where articular cartilage is accessible, it appears as a thin low-reflectivity layer immediately overlying cortical/subchondral bone (Figure 13.22, on DVD). When fluid overlies the cartilage, a thin line of increased reflectivity is typically shown (Figure 13.23). Although articular hyaline cartilage is lower in reflectivity, many joints also contain structures formed of fibro-cartilage, such as the menisci in the knee or the labrum of the acetabulum or glenoid. Fibro-cartilaginous structures are highly reflective (Figure 13.24). Fluid within joints may be detectable normally in small quantities, depending upon the joint, but when associated

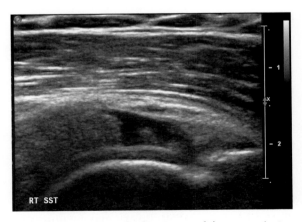

Figure 13.23 Longitudinal US image of the supraspinatus tendon demonstrating fluid within a full thickness tear. Note the increased reflectivity of the articular cartilage surface where it is covered by fluid rather than tendon.

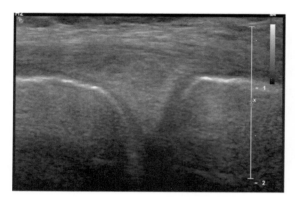

Figure 13.24 US image of the medial meniscus, shown as a highly reflective triangle.

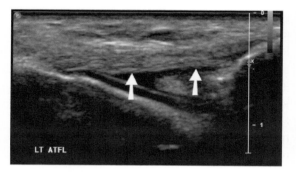

Figure 13.27 US image of the anterior talofibular ligament (arrows).

with capsular distension it is almost always pathological. Joint fluid is typically very low in reflectivity in normal cases (Figure 13.25, on DVD). Highly reflective fluid collections can be observed in pathological cases, and whilst not pathognomonic of infection/inflammation, are undoubtedly commonly associated with these conditions and aspiration is often required. The capsular and ligamentous tissues supporting a joint are readily detectable as relatively high-reflectivity tissue. The thin layer of synovium which lines the joint capsule is not identifiable when normal, but thickened synovium is readily identified on ultrasound when surrounded by joint fluid (Figure 13.26, on DVD). It is frequently difficult to identify ligaments as discrete structures from surrounding tissue, although this is possible in certain situations, particularly when the ligament is not fused with the remainder of the joint capsule. Common examples are the anterior talofibular ligament at the ankle (Figure 13.27) and the acromioclavicular ligament in the shoulder.

Bursae are other structures which assist musculoskeletal movement and comprise a sack-like capsule containing a small amount of fluid (Figure 13.28, on DVD). Bursae may be normally present or can develop in response to friction. Some bursae communicate with adjacent joints. Some bursae are located between bone and overlying skin

(subcutaneous) and others are located deep to fascia, typically separating bone from other structures such as tendon or ligament. Bursae are typically lined by a thin layer of synovial tissue which cannot be distinguished from the relatively reflective bursal capsule. If the amount of fluid present is minimal, the bursal walls are approximated and the intersection appears as a thin line of reduced reflectivity. Frequently, a small amount of fluid is present and the bursa is easier to identify.

Ultrasound in muscle, joint and other soft tissue injury

This section discusses the ultrasound appearances of pathology which may be encountered in the musculoskeletal system. It is by necessity a relatively brief overview, and readers wishing to develop skills further are referred to a number of excellent textbooks at the end of the chapter. It should be noted that the learning curve for developing comprehensive skills in musculoskeletal ultrasound is long and practitioners should ensure they have appropriate training and an experienced mentor to whom they can refer.

Muscle injury

This section will be divided into discussions of acute injury, chronic injury and complications.

Acute muscle injuries may be direct or indirect. Indirect muscle injuries are extremely common sporting injuries at all levels of activity. The lower limb is most commonly affected.

Indirect muscle injury

DELAYED ONSET MUSCLE SORENESS (DOMS)

DOMS is manifest by diffuse muscle pain occurring typically 12–24 h after unaccustomed strenuous activity. It usually resolves over several days without requiring treatment and imaging is rarely necessary. When performed, ultrasound is usually normal, although MRI may show features of multifocal muscle edema.

Muscle strain

Muscle strains are the result of excessive force applied by the muscle itself rather than an external insult applied to the muscle. Muscles which cross more than one joint are more susceptible and therefore, in the lower limb, hamstring and rectus femoris strains are more common than those affecting the vasti or adductor muscle groups. Muscle strains frequently affect the vulnerable myotendinous junction. Muscle strains are manifest by tearing at this site with hemorrhage followed by an edematous and inflammatory response. Healing subsequently occurs with the time required variable depending on the severity of the initial injury. Muscle strains are distinguished from DOMS on clinical grounds, with an immediate onset of pain and a focal nature allowing some, although not necessarily totally accurate, localization. Muscle strains are clinically graded between 1 and 3, with the latter indicating a complete muscle tear and no detectable residual function. On ultrasound, grade 1 muscle strains may be undetectable or show very minor areas of hemorrhage and disturbance of normal muscle architecture (Figure 13.29, on DVD). Injuries may be categorized as grade 1 provided no more than 5% of muscle function is lost clinically and on ultrasound, provided that no more than 5% of muscle volume is affected.

Muscle strains are categorized as grade 2 where the extent of injury is above 5% but not 100% of the muscle. Grade 2 tears typically show more extensive intramuscular fluid or hemorrhage (Figure 13.30, on DVD), the extent of which can be underestimated if heavy compression is applied with the probe, as noted earlier in the chapter. Sonographers should vary the amount of pressure in order to avoid this pitfall. The use of ultrasound's dynamic advantages, by scanning the muscle both in relaxation and contraction, is a useful maneuver to help assess the extent of the injury. Grade 3 injuries are complete tears with retraction of the muscle away from the site of the injury (Figure 13.31, on DVD). Retraction is further emphasized by scanning as the patient contracts the muscle. The retracted muscle belly is frequently surrounded by hyporeflective hematoma/fluid known as the "bell-clapper" sign, although this appearance may also be observed in partial/grade 2 injuries.

Direct muscle injuries

Direct muscle injuries may occur as a result of blunt or penetrating trauma. Blunt traumatic injuries are termed muscle contusions, whilst penetrating injuries are termed muscle lacerations.

MUSCLE CONTUSION

Muscle contusions are frequently observed when muscle is compressed against underlying bone and the lower limb is more commonly affected. Early after the injury, ultrasound demonstrates a swollen area of part or occasionally a complete muscle with increased reflectivity. After approximately 48 h, intramuscular hematoma organizes and becomes better defined. Over subsequent days/weeks, low-reflectivity hematoma gradually dissipates from the periphery and the muscle appearances return to normal. Extensive contusional injuries may progress to large

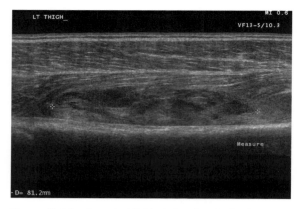

Figure 13.32 Extended field of view longitudinal US image demonstrating a large hematoma within the vastus intermedius muscle belly. The overlying rectus femoris muscle appears normal.

intramuscular hematomas (Figure 13.32), scarring or less frequently myositis ossificans.

MUSCLE LACERATION

Penetrating muscle injuries are less common than contusions or indirect trauma. Lacerations are typically linear and frequently heal with a residual scar.

Chronic injuries and complications

Many muscle injuries heal successfully with no residual scar or defect. Scarring may occur in severe muscle injury and is particularly prevalent following laceration. The scar may be asymptomatic, but will restrict muscle function and may affect an athlete's future performance. On ultrasound, the scar shows increased reflectivity typically with indrawing of surrounding muscle tissue, and dynamic scanning demonstrates a relatively rigid area of tissue. Because of the prevalence of muscle injuries in the myotendinous junction area (Figure 13.33, on DVD), a scar is particularly common in this region.

Muscle atrophy

Following grade 3 muscle strains in which the muscle is completely torn, failure of subsequent healing results in disuse atrophy of the muscle belly, loss of volume and diffuse increased reflectivity secondary to transformation of muscle tissue to fat.

Myositis ossificans

Myositis ossificans refers to the failure of resorption of a muscle hematoma which subsequently proceeds to ossify from the periphery. A history of previous injury is not always obtained. Early peripheral calcification may be detectable at the edges of a hematoma within two months and progressively matures (Figure 13.34, on DVD). Small ossified lesions may be asymptomatic, but larger masses often cause excessive pain and swelling early in the course of the disease and, when mature, a hard swelling may be palpable in some cases. This may be surgically removed, but intervention is best delayed until full maturity has occurred. In some cases, medical treatment with biphosphonates is used. Ultrasound is very sensitive to the early peripheral calcification/ossification and can demonstrate changes earlier than they are visible on X-ray. MRI of myositis ossificans can be easily misinterpreted as showing a soft tissue sarcoma, and this is a particular risk when there is no history of previous injury. Ultrasound cannot, however, image deep to well-established soft tissue calcification, and in these circumstances, differentiation of myositis ossificans from bone lesions such as osteochondroma or parosteal osteosarcoma is extremely difficult. X-ray or CT may be necessary in these cases (Figure 13.35).

Muscle hernia

The term muscle hernia refers to the bulge of muscle tissue through an area of weakness in its peripheral fascia or epimysium. Patients may present with local pain and frequently a swelling which is detectable when the muscle is contracted but absent on relaxation. MRI of the area is usually normal, as imaging is performed in relaxation and patients may

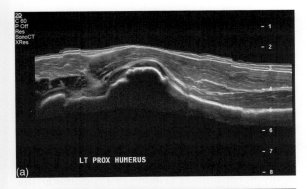

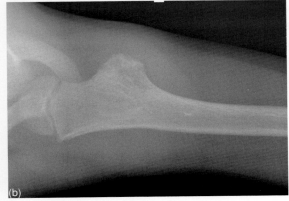

Figure 13.35 Longitudinal extended field of view US image (a) and radiograph (b) demonstrating an osteochondroma of the proximal left humerus.

become frustrated by the lack of a diagnosis under such circumstances. Muscle hernias are particularly common in the lower leg, particularly tibialis anterior (Figure 13.36, on DVD), but may be demonstrated in other areas such as the thigh or forearm (Figure 13.37, on DVD). Muscle hernias may be readily detectable by simply contracting the affected muscle, but in some situations only become apparent after a period of exercise. Because pressure from the ultrasound probe can easily "relocate" the protruding muscle tissue, applying a thick layer of gel to the area and avoiding direct contact between the probe and the skin can be extremely useful. Careful ultrasound technique allows detection of the fascial defect as an interruption in the usually high-reflective fascial stripe.

Tendon pathology

Tendon injuries generally affect an older (typically middle-aged) patient group than injuries of muscle. Although the term "tendinitis" is commonly used, this is best avoided unless the condition is clearly inflammatory. "Tendinosis" or "tendinopathy" are more typically used by musculoskeletal imagers. Either term refers to the typically degenerative process which occurs due to what is frequently considered an overuse type injury. The most commonly affected tendon is the Achilles, and the development of Achilles tendinopathy is also influenced by factors such as patient body habitus and hyperpronation of the foot. When severe, tendinopathy progresses to macroscopic partial tear or cyst formation within the tendon substance or even complete rupture. In addition to pathology of the tendon itself, the periphery may also be affected – in tendons with a synovial sheath, this is referred to as tenosynovitis, and in tendons lacking a sheath, paratenonitis.

The ultrasound features of tendinopathy are of tendon swelling combined with a reduction in reflectivity. In the Achilles tendon, the swelling is typically fusiform in shape (Figure 13.38, on DVD), and the reduction in reflectivity may be patchy. In the Achilles tendon and patellar tendon, tendinopathy is usually easy to identify by scanning along the long axis of the tendon. In areas of more complex anatomy such as the ankle and wrist, it is usually more helpful to begin the examination with a transverse orientation in order to correctly identify the tendon of interest. This is particularly so at the ankle, where the tendons change direction as they pass around the malleoli and imaging in the longitudinal axis is difficult. The features of tendinopathy can nevertheless be observed in both the longitudinal and transverse orientations (Figure 13.39, on DVD). Applying Doppler to the area of affected tendon frequently reveals increased blood flow in the form of slender branching vessels mainly related to the anterior/deep surface of the tendon (Figure 13.40, on DVD). The significance of this neovascularization is unknown. Vessels are well demonstrated by color or power Doppler, and wave form interrogation is possible with pulsed/spectral Doppler. This may reveal either venous or arterial wave form patterns.

In tendons without synovial sheaths such as the Achilles, tendinopathy is frequently accompanied by changes in the surrounding loose connective tissue, termed paratenonopathy or paratenonitis. These changes can be inferred by the presence of increased vascularity within the paratenon tissue and particularly by thickening and the reduction in reflectivity of the normally thin and highly reflective epitendineum (Figure 13.41, on DVD). Tendons with synovial sheaths, when affected by a tendinopathic process, frequently also demonstrate increased tendon sheath fluid and thickening of the synovial lining which may be irregular and show increased vascularity within the abnormal synovial tissue (Figure 13.42, on DVD). A small amount of fluid may be normally observed within the tendon sheaths at the ankle, although the amount considered to be within normal limits varies between different tendons (Figure 13.43, on DVD). Around the wrist, it is unusual to observe tendon sheath fluid collections in normal cases.

The changes of tenosynovitis may be observed surrounding an otherwise normal tendon, typically in conditions such as rheumatoid arthritis, where progress to subsequent tendon changes and even rupture may occur, or secondary to overuse (Figure 13.44, on DVD). At the wrist, tenosynovitis affecting the first extensor compartment tendons (abductor pollicis longus and extensor pollicis brevis) is known as de Quervains or stenosing tenosynovitis. In this form of tendon sheath disorder, fluid is frequently, although not always, absent and the disorder is manifested by thickening of the tendon sheath (Figure 13.45, on DVD).

Advanced tendon disorders

Tendinopathic changes have a spectrum of appearances and severities, typically categorized mainly by the extent of tendon involvement and the maximal thickness achieved. As further disease progression occurs, macroscopic partial tears or complete rupture of the tendon occurs, and the tendon may then demonstrate focal areas of intensely low reflectivity (Figure 13.46, on DVD) or become focally much thinner (Figure 13.47, on DVD). It can be difficult to distinguish precisely when severe tendinopathy becomes a partial tear, particularly in the Achilles and patellar tendons, where areas of focal reduced reflectivity are surrounded by more normal-appearing tendon tissue. In tibialis posterior, the presence of a partial tear changes the clinical grading score and influences management.

Complete tendon rupture results in clinical loss of function of the affected muscle and, in certain cases, typically tendon disorders related to inflammatory arthritis, can result in symptom reduction, although more commonly, the loss of function causes new clinical problems, such as the inability to toe rise following Achilles rupture. In tendons with a synovial sheath lining, rupture results in retraction of the tendon and muscle belly away from the site of the tear. The sheath may then be observed to contain fluid but no tendon (Figure 13.48, on DVD), or may collapse and be difficult to detect (Figure 13.49). In tendons with a surrounding paratenon, this may also tear, and the gap between the free ends of the tendon is typically filled by a combination of hemorrhage, prolapsed paratenon and surrounding fat (Figure 13.50, on DVD). In the Achilles tendon, dynamic ultrasound is of great value in assessing whether the free ends of the tear are in contact, typically when the ankle is plantar flexed. When contact is observed, conservative management may be possible, whereas surgical repair is necessary if the ends remain widely separated.

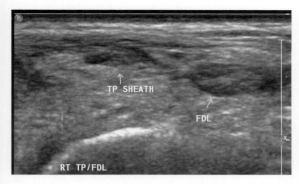

Figure 13.49 US image following rupture of the tibialis posterior (TP) tendon tear demonstrating an empty sheath with slightly thickened walls. The adjacent flexor digitorum longus (FDL) tendon appears normal.

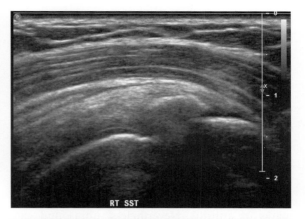

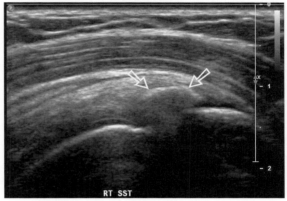

Figure 13.51 US image of the supraspinatus tendon which contains a large deposit of calcific tendonitis (arrows). Note the acoustic shadowing deep to the deposit obscuring the surface of the greater tuberosity.

A distinct cause of tendon symptoms and abnormalities on ultrasound is calcific tendonitis, a process where deposition of calcium hydroxapatite within the tendon causes intense pain. The deposits can be observed within the tendon substance on radiographs and ultrasound (Figure 13.51). The latter demonstrates appearances similar to those of a gallstone, with a curved, highly reflective lesion and posterior acoustic shadowing obscuring deeper structures. Ultrasound can be used to guide aspiration or injection of the deposits.

Ligament injury

The role of ultrasound in evaluating ligaments is rather more limited. Ligaments appear generally similar to tendons on ultrasound when the ultrasound beam is perpendicular to the long axis of the ligament (Figure 13.52, on DVD). Ligaments are generally shorter and frequently have an orientation such that it is difficult to adequately evaluate them with ultrasound. Examples of this are the calcaneo-fibular and posterior talo-fibular ligaments, both of which are difficult to reliably trace from origin to insertion. The anterior talo-fibular ligament, the most anterior and vulnerable of the lateral ankle ligament complex, is more reliably demonstrated (Figure 13.53, on DVD), but even

here it can be difficult to assess the severity of any injury. At the knee, the medial collateral ligament is easily observed (Figure 13.54, on DVD) and the severity of injury can usually be accurately assessed. The pitfall here is of "search satisfaction". Whilst knee collateral ligament injuries can be diagnosed, they are commonly associated with other knee pathology such as cruciate or meniscal tears, or articular surface damage, which cannot be accurately diagnosed or even reliably observed with ultrasound, and sonographers must always be aware of the limitations of the technique in order to avoid missing potentially significant injuries. On ultrasound, ligaments when injured behave in a

189

similar manner to tendons, demonstrating thickening and a reduction in reflectivity.

Joint and bursal abnormalities

Ultrasound is by no means the investigation of choice when selecting an imaging modality to assess a patient with joint disease. Ultrasound cannot access the entire articular surface of any joint, nor can it demonstrate bone marrow edema or other features within bone, such as subchondral cyst formation or sclerosis, which can be hallmarks of arthritis. Nevertheless, ultrasound can successfully demonstrate distension of a joint by either fluid (Figure 13.55, on DVD) or solid material (Figure 13.56, on DVD), since most joints allow at least some ultrasound access, and even those where it is limited usually have ultrasound-accessible recesses which will fill with synovial fluid or thickening. It is therefore important for sonographers to have some familiarity with the capsular boundaries of joints they wish to scan, and to understand the difference between communicating and non-communicating bursae – the former serving as potential spaces into which tense joint effusions may decompress. Examples of communicating bursae include a Baker's cyst at the knee (Figure 13.57, on DVD) and the ilio-psoas bursa at the hip, communicating with the joint in approximately 20% of adults (Figure 13.58, on DVD). Communicating bursae are thought to develop with age and are rarely encountered in children. Certain bursae only communicate with a joint under pathological circumstances – for example, the subacromial/subdeltoid bursa of the shoulder is separated from the gleno-humeral joint by the rotator cuff tendon and communication is only established by a full thickness rotator cuff tear (Figure 13.59, on DVD).

A joint effusion is a non-specific finding indicating joint pathology, but may be seen in a range of processes such as osteoarthritis, joint inflammation, avascular necrosis, infection, or tumor. Although ultrasound may be unable to reliably distinguish the cause of the effusion, it is extremely sensitive at detecting even small amounts of joint fluid, and is of great value in situations such as the assessment of the painful pediatric hip. Hip joint effusion is detected on ultrasound when fluid accumulates in the capsular recess over the femoral neck (Figure 13.60, on DVD). The distance between the cortical surface of the neck and the overlying capsule is measured, and a depth of fluid greater than 3 mm or an asymmetry of greater than 2 mm between the normal and abnormal sides is considered significant. Ultrasound can also assist or guide subsequent aspiration of fluid to test for infective organisms. The major differential diagnosis of septic arthritis of the hip in a child is transient synovitis. Fluid obtained in this condition is typically serous or mildly blood-stained. Infected joint fluid may be purulent, but ultrasound is unable to reliably distinguish the nature of fluid, and aspiration cannot, therefore, be avoided. Serous joint fluid is typically anechoic on ultrasound, and intra-articular pus typically shows fluid of increased reflectivity, but exceptions to both of these statements are not infrequently encountered. Hemorrhagic joint effusions in trauma (Figure 13.61, on DVD) may be diagnosed when the complex fluid contains solid blood clot, but clearly the history is vital. Other causes of complex joint fluid collections would include chronic inflammatory arthritis, pigmented villonodular synovitis and synovial osteochondromatosis, in all cases demonstrating a combination of complex effusion and solid intra-articular or synovial material. Such cases will usually require specialist referral and further imaging.

Ultrasound is of great value in distinguishing between joint distension due to effusion or synovitis. This distinction cannot be made on X-ray (Figure 13.62, on DVD), and MRI frequently requires intravenous contrast enhancement to

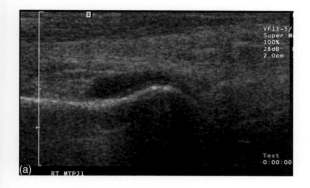

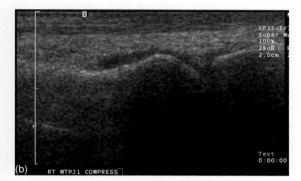

Figure 13.64 Longitudinal US images of the dorsal aspect of the right first metatarsophalangeal joint before (a) and after (b) compression. The second image shows displacement of the joint effusion shown on the first image.

confirm the presence of thickened, vascularized synovium (Figure 13.63, on DVD). On ultrasound, distinction is readily made by the simple application of pressure with a probe which will displace fluid but not solid, thickened joint lining (Figure 13.64). When an anechoic effusion is present, synovial thickening may be outlined by fluid. The use of Doppler readily allows an assessment of synovial vascularity (Figure 13.65, on DVD). When a joint effusion is present and fluid is required to test for infection or a crystal deposition arthritis, ultrasound guidance has been shown to increase the yield from percutaneous aspiration (Balint). Ultrasound has also been shown to be more sensitive than plain radiographs in the detection of erosions due to inflammatory arthritis (Wakefield).

Ultrasound of fluid and solid mass lesion

Ultrasound is a highly useful imaging modality in the evaluation of a wide range of soft tissue masses, as it readily distinguishes solid and cystic masses, can assess internal vascularity, and allows a dynamic assessment of the compressibility of the lesion and its relationship to surrounding structures. Ultrasound can make a definitive diagnosis in a large number of cases, and can obviate the need for ongoing referral to a sarcoma center, MRI and biopsy, provided the sonographer is familiar with the ultrasound of soft tissue lesions. Nevertheless, there are some cases where suspicion of a malignant lesion is high and further imaging and biopsy will be required. In other lesions, ultrasound cannot determine a precise diagnosis and here, a sensible approach based on the clinical history and patient's wishes is required. Small, superficial solid masses which show no suspicious ultrasound features and are not painful or rapidly enlarging can usually be followed up, possibly with a repeat examination, provided the patient is happy with this strategy. Those soft tissue masses which show features suspicious of a sarcoma should be referred directly to a sarcoma center under NICE guidance. These features are of a lump which is:

(1) greater than 5 cm in diameter,
(2) deep to the fascia, fixed or immobile,
(3) increasing in size,
(4) painful, and
(5) a recurrence after a previous sarcoma excision.

An exhaustive description of the ultrasound features of all fluid and soft tissue masses is beyond the scope of this chapter, and a logical approach to the evaluation of a lump will be described.

Initially the sonographer should take a brief history and examine the lump as part of the normal process of greeting the patient and putting them at ease in the correct position for the examination. This often yields valuable information regarding the duration of symptoms, but sonographers should bear in mind that soft tissue sarcoma may be painless and patients may play down symptoms because of anxiety. The first step is to identify the patient's perceived lump on ultrasound. Probe selection is important here since deep lumps may be beyond the reach of some very high-frequency transducers, whilst very superficial small lumps may be difficult to observe when a lower-frequency probe is used. It is important to establish a definite link between what is being palpated clinically and any suspected "lump" observed on the ultrasound screen. A lump which is due to muscle hernias may not be visible when the affected muscle is relaxed, and this information could also be sought if there is any difficulty in identifying a focal lesion. Once the lump has been identified, it is important to take note of its depth, relation to the deep fascia, size, the presence or absence of vascularity on Doppler, and whether it appears to be fully or partially fluid. Fluid masses may be bursal, ganglions, vascular structures such as varices or aneurysms or, if closely associated with a fibro-cartilaginous joint structure such as a meniscus or labrum, a meniscal or paralabral cyst due to extravazation of synovial fluid through a tear and into the surrounding connective tissue. The sonographer should be aware of the location of the common bursae encountered in ultrasound examinations (such as the subacromial/subdeltoid bursa in the shoulder, the bicipito-radial and olecranon bursae at the elbow, the ilio-psoas bursa at the hip, the retro-calcaneal bursa on the posterior aspect of the ankle and the numerous bursae which may be encountered around the knee). Some bursae may form due to the effects of pressure, and in unusual locations it is important to consider the possibility of an underlying bone prominence such as an osteochondroma. Bursae may be lined by thickened synovial tissue (Figure 13.65, on

DVD) and if inflamed show vascularity on Doppler studies. On occasions, appearances may be alarming, and if unable to exclude a soft tissue sarcoma, the sonographer should always err on the side of caution and refer the patient for further assessment.

Ganglia (Figure 13.66, on DVD) are common soft tissue lesions which are cystic but frequently contain highly viscous material and may be so firm that they mimic bone lesions. It is common for such a patient to be initially referred for a radiograph to assess a bony lump. Ganglia are distinct from soft tissue synovial cysts pathologically as they lack a synovial membrane lining, but this distinction cannot be made on ultrasound. Ganglia may arise de novo or can be due to synovial fluid escaping from a joint or tendon sheath, in which case the sonographer may be able to demonstrate communication between the ganglion and the feeding structure. Ganglia are commonly encountered in the foot and carpal areas.

Vascular cystic structures (Figure 13.67, on DVD) are usually easy to diagnose by a combination of their Doppler patterns and the identification of a usually large vessel entering or exiting the lesion. Meniscal and paralabral cysts (Figure 13.68, on DVD) should be suspected whenever a fluid collection is identified outside a joint but close to a labrum or meniscus. It is frequently difficult to identify the fibro-cartilage tear, but in most cases this would be closely associated with the cyst. In the knee, cysts related to tears of the lateral meniscus generally form at the immediate periphery of the meniscus within loose connective tissue. On the medial side, the periphery of the middle third of the meniscus is tightly bound to the overlying medial collateral ligament and here there is no space for fluid to accumulate. Fluid tracking through tears of the middle third of the medial meniscus therefore has to travel further before it reaches a point where cyst formation can occur, and generally a slender track of fluid proceeds either anteriorly or

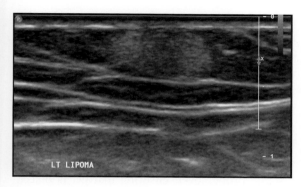

Figure 13.70 US image of a simple subcutaneous lipoma shown as an ovoid lesion of slightly higher reflectivity than surrounding fat.

posteriorly to the margin of the ligament before the cyst forms. Meniscal and paralabral cysts cannot be treated successfully by aspiration or excision without treating the underlying tear and therefore this is an important diagnosis to establish.

Solid mass lesions which are large, low in reflectivity, lobulated and show high, particularly disordered vascularity, are highly suspicious (Figure 13.69, on DVD), and must be treated as presumed soft tissue sarcoma until proven otherwise. Such lesions are generally firm and cannot be compressed by the application of pressure from the probe. Masses composed of fat (Figure 13.70) are generally readily compressible, particularly when superficial to the fascia. When assessing compressibility, it is important to ensure that one is not already pressing firmly enough to have deformed the natural shape of a lesion, and it is often most useful to consciously reduce pressure with the probe initially almost to the point where contact with the skin surface is lost, as this may demonstrate a naturally much more rounded lesion than was previously suspected. This maneuver can be assisted by applying a layer of thick ultrasound jelly which can act as a "stand-off". Other features to note in the evaluation of soft tissue masses are the shape of the lesion, elongated or spindle-shaped lesions being less suspicious, the relationship of the lesion to a

neurovascular bundle, and particularly the identification of an entering or exiting nerve, which is highly suggestive that the lesion is a nerve sheath tumor, internal areas of cystic change, calcification or other highly reflective materials. Cystic change within the lesion is a non-specific feature which can indicate necrosis of the tumor, but can also be observed in vascular malformations or hemangiomas because of the presence of blood-filled venous lakes. These may drain with compression from the probe or by direct elevation of the affected limp. Rarely, fluid levels may be observed within such cysts, highly suggestive of the presence of hemorrhagic spaces (Figure 13.67, on DVD). Once again, hemangiomas can cause this appearance. The commonest soft tissue sarcoma to demonstrate internal fluid levels is a synovial sarcoma.

Calcification can be observed within a wide range of soft tissue masses including fat necrosis, pilomatrixoma, and synovial sarcoma (once again this is the commonest soft tissue sarcoma to display this feature), or if the calcifications are well-defined and round, they may be phleboliths within a hemangioma. Calcification of the periphery of a lesion is suggestive of myositis ossificans (Figure 13.34, on DVD), which may demonstrate alarming vascularity on Doppler. Linear foci of high reflectivity may be observed in foreign body granulomas, particularly due to the presence of glass or thorn (Figure 13.71, on DVD). Glass fragments are generally radio-opaque and usually diagnosed radiographically, but plant material is radiolucent and often incites a surrounding inflammatory response which is relatively low in reflectivity and outlines the plant or thorn. Foreign bodies may also enter tendon sheaths in the extremities. In addition to causing an inflammatory or infective tenosynovitis, the foreign body may migrate along the length of the sheath and ultrasound is best performed immediately prior to removal in order to identify the current position of the fragment.

Interventional musculoskeletal ultrasound

The dynamic nature of ultrasound and its excellent resolution of soft tissue structures makes it an ideal modality for assisting with a wide range of percutaneous procedures. Ultrasound may be used simply to assist aspiration – for example, in the infant hip effusion, where it is used to confirm the preferred needle entry point, direction and depth to which the needle should be inserted in order to access the fluid collection of interest. In this situation, the probe is not used to visualize the needle but simply used prior to skin preparation and anesthesia. Although ultrasound assistance undoubtedly has a role, in most cases, ultrasound guidance is preferable – here the needle is observed and directed to the target as visualized on the ultrasound screen. Ultrasound guidance is preferable for biopsy procedures to ensure that the best tissue is obtained, and for diagnostic and therapeutic local anesthetic and steroid injections to ensure that the active agent is correctly delivered to the intended target. Ultrasound-guided techniques frequently require practitioners who are used to performing such injections without ultrasound to rethink their approach, since the most direct route between skin and target rarely allows ideal visualization of the needle. A more oblique approach is required (Figure 13.72, on DVD) in most cases to allow the ultrasound beam to intersect the needle at a more preferable angle (typically between 60° and 90° to the long axis of the needle) and frequently to permit space for both probe and needle to be positioned on the skin. It is important to allow time to consider the optimum positioning of the needle entry point and probe, since careful attention to this decision can save considerable time and difficulty later in the procedure. The route between skin entry point and target must be planned such that it avoids damage to other important structures. The entry point can be marked with an indelible

pen, but can be perfectly satisfactorily defined by pressure from a firm structure such as a paper clip or the open end of a plastic needle cover. Once the route has been determined, ultrasound gel is cleared from the area and the entry point sterilised. Formal preparation is preferable for procedures involving puncture of a joint, whilst sterile skin swabs may be used for other soft tissue injections and aspirations. The surface of the probe can be covered with a sterile probe cover, ensuring that gel is placed within the cover in contact with the transducer surface. Sterile ultrasound jelly may then be applied to the skin, ensuring satisfactory visualization. The needle is then introduced into the skin and identified on the ultrasound image by coordination of the needle and probe. Needle guides, fixing the needle to the side of the probe, with a variable or fixed angle are available, but these are frequently rather restrictive and do not allow much adjustment once the procedure is underway. Most radiologists prefer to hold the needle and probe independently, although some skill is required in ensuring that the needle is well demonstrated. Ideally, the probe should be orientated such that the long axis of the needle lies within the scan plane and both shaft and tip are visualized. If only part of the shaft is demonstrated, then the sonographer cannot be sure of the location of the needle tip, and the needle should not be advanced further until the tip is relocalized. The needle shaft may be identified by turning the probe through 90°, but, once again, it is difficult to be certain of the location of the needle tip in this situation and this technique should only be used by experienced practitioners. Once needle, target and probe are satisfactorily aligned, the needle may be advanced and adjustments made to its direction if necessary. In addition to aspirations, injections and biopsies, ultrasound can be used to deploy a guide wire within a tumor to aid surgical localizations (Figure 13.73, on DVD). In the case of soft tissue sarcoma, biopsy and wire localization should only be performed after consultation with the surgeon who will perform the definitive excision to ensure that surgical options are not compromised by contamination of soft tissue compartments which would be otherwise preserved.

Summary

This chapter has discussed issues specific to ultrasound of the musculoskeletal system, the normal appearances of soft tissue and other structures encountered, and the range of pathologies which may be investigated and in some cases potentially treated by ultrasound-guided techniques. Musculoskeletal ultrasound is a distinct area of specialization in its own right and has a steep learning curve. Although this chapter will hopefully act as a source of useful information and direction for further, more advanced, reading, it should be remembered that any sonographer wishing to develop skills in this area should train appropriately under the guidance of an already experienced practitioner, and should have clear documentary evidence of the training they have undertaken. Outside of the environment of a normal radiology department, consideration should be given also to issues regarding the storage and retention of ultrasound images and reports for further reference.

FURTHER READING

Balint PV, Kane D, Hunter J, et al. Ultrasound guided versus conventional joint and soft tissue fluid aspiration in rheumatology practice: a pilot study. *Journal of Rheumatology* 2000;29:2209–13.

Wakefield RJ, Gibbon WW, O'Connor P. High resolution ultrasound: a superior method to radiography for detecting cortical bone erosions in rheumatoid arthritis (abstract). *British Journal of Rheumatology* 1998;7:S197.

van Holsbeeck M. *Musculoskeletal Ultrasound*. 2nd edn. Philadelphia: Mosby, 2001.

McNally EG. *Practical Musculoskeletal Ultrasound*. Churchill Livingstone, 2004.

National Institute for Health and Clinical Excellence Guideline CG27. Referral for suspected cancer, 2005, p. 90.

Index